Psychological Impact of Behaviour Restrictions During the Pandemic

This volume examines the undesirable or harmful cognitive, emotional and behavioural side-effects of COVID-19 and of the behavioural restrictions imposed by governments on their populations during the pandemic.

Societal "lockdowns" and other intervening behavioural restrictions, built significantly around social isolation, used by governments to control the spread of COVID-19 disrupted the lives of most people. There were economic costs for many as workplaces closed down, as well as severe stresses on friendships and romantic relationships, an increase in instances of abuse and domestic violence, and concerns about people drinking too much alcohol or gambling too much as compensatory behaviours. Understanding which people were at risk, and in what ways, could teach important lessons for the future. Presenting a timely review of the most recent international research and evidence, author Barrie Gunter assesses the major collateral, psychological side-effects of the pandemic. Looking forward, Gunter also considers how new models might be developed that take into account not just the need to halt the spread of a new virus, but also minimise collateral damage which could be every bit as severe in both the short term and long term.

Identifying and analysing the nature and severity of collateral side-effects of pandemic-related behaviour restrictions, this is essential reading for students and researchers in psychology, public health and medical sciences and policymakers assessing government strategies, responses and performance.

Barrie Gunter is an Emeritus Professor in Media at the University of Leicester, United Kingdom. A psychologist by training, he has published more than 80 books on a range of media, marketing, business, leisure and psychology topics.

Psychological Impact of Behaviour Restrictions During the Pandemic

Lessons from COVID-19

Barrie Gunter

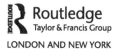

Routledge
Taylor & Francis Group

LONDON AND NEW YORK

Cover image: Getty

First published 2022
by Routledge
4 Park Square, Milton Park, Abingdon, Oxon OX14 4RN

and by Routledge
605 Third Avenue, New York, NY 10158

Routledge is an imprint of the Taylor & Francis Group, an informa business

British Library Cataloguing-in-Publication Data
A catalogue record for this book is available from the British Library

Library of Congress Cataloging-in-Publication Data
Names: Gunter, Barrie, author.
Title: Psychological impact of behaviour restrictions during the pandemic :
lessons from COVID-19 / Barrie Gunter.
Description: Abingdon, Oxon ; New York, NY : Routledge, 2022. | Includes
bibliographical references and index. | Summary: "This volume examines the
undesirable or harmful cognitive, emotional and behavioural side-effects of
COVID-19, and of the behavioural restrictions imposed by governments on
their populations during the pandemic"-- Provided by publisher.
Identifiers: LCCN 2022013169 (print) | LCCN 2022013170 (ebook) |
ISBN 9781032228280 (v. 2 ; hardback) | ISBN 9781032228259
(v. 2 ; paperback) | ISBN 9781003274377 (v. 2 ; ebook)
Subjects: LCSH: Behavior modification. | Health promotion. |
COVID-19 Pandemic, 2020---Psychological aspects.
Classification: LCC BF637.B4 G85 2022 (print) | LCC BF637.B4 (ebook) |
DDC 153.8/5--dc23/eng/20220506
LC record available at https://lccn.loc.gov/2022013169
LC ebook record available at https://lccn.loc.gov/2022013170

ISBN: 978-1-032-22828-0 (hbk)
ISBN: 978-1-032-22825-9 (pbk)
ISBN: 978-1-003-27437-7 (ebk)

DOI: 10.4324/9781003274377

Typeset in Sabon
by MPS Limited, Dehradun

Contents

Chapter 1

The COVID-19 Pandemic: Hindsight and Foresight

When first identified, the *novel* coronavirus, COVID-19, was a completely new virus about which little was known and for which there were no established preventative or treatment-related medical interventions. Being new also meant that human beings had no acquired immunity to it, although a few may have had some serendipitous natural immunity. Despite this particular virus being new, the family of coronaviruses was not unknown. Yet, the distinctive characteristics of this specific coronavirus meant the whole world was confronted with a steep learning curve in trying rapidly to understand more about its structure, infectivity, symptoms and potential to cause death. It also meant leaning heavily on non-medical or non-pharmaceutical interventions, initially, to bring it under control as it spread rapidly around the globe.

In turning to non-pharmaceutical measures, which were based on recommended personal hygiene and protection behaviours and limited social contact with other people, restrictions were introduced that brought sweeping changes to people's lives. It was quickly apparent also that these so-called "protective" measures could cause considerable collateral damage of their own to individuals, families, businesses and services. The enforced closure of many physical spaces in which people would normally intermingle was implemented by many national governments because there were doubts that reliance on the public's voluntary compliance would not deliver the desired results.

Mistakes were made. Some governments closed down too late. Others did not close down sufficiently or for long enough. Some failed to get to grips with the types of physical spaces that posed the greatest risk of infection spread. Many defended their decisions by reminding everyone that this was a major crisis involving a new virus and its impact was being felt across the world on an unprecedented scale. Too little was therefore known to provide detailed strategic guidance about how best to tackle the rapid spread of highly infectious disease The defence of "benefit of hindsight" did not always ring true, however, given previous warnings governments had received from public health experts and scientists about the risks of major pandemics

DOI: 10.4324/9781003274377-1

(Henig, 2020, 9th April). To be clear, pandemics were known about and had been recently experienced, even during the 21st century. The deployment of non-pharmaceutical interventions was also established practice for dealing with pandemics until effective medical treatments were available.

Advance Warnings

In August 2010, the Director General of the World Health Organization (WHO) warned, as the world recovered from H1N1 pandemic, that pandemics were unpredictable and could have unexpected impacts. The H1N1 pandemic had been relatively mild, but it could have turned out differently. The WHO issued advice however that people should continue to observe good personal hand and respiratory hygiene, take up vaccines when offered and observe other locally recommended practices designed to control the spread of the virus (WHO, 2010, August).

In a widely viewed TED Talk delivered in March 2015, five years before the onset of the 2020 novel coronavirus pandemic, the entrepreneur turned philanthropist Bill Gates issued a warning that a global pandemic would soon occur for which the world was ill-prepared. It would infect hundreds of millions and kill millions and place health systems under considerable strain. In the absence of pharmaceutical protection from vaccines and therapeutic drugs at the outset, societies would need to deploy a range of non-pharmaceutical measures and this would entail the suspension of normal activities and extensive shutdown of their workforces costing the global economy trillions of dollars. Gates offered some insights into how governments and the international community could prepare, but few did (Gates, 2015).

Ralph Baric, an epidemiologist at the University of North Carolina, warned about the risks of pandemic outbreaks in papers published in *Nature* in 2015 and *PNAS* in 2016. His warnings were especially poignant and prescient given its references to viruses circulating in bat populations that might prove to be zoonotic. Baric and his co-workers identified further variants of the severe acute respiratory syndrome coronavirus (SARS-CoV) and the Middle East respiratory syndrome (MERS-CoV) coronavirus could emerge. In fact, a bat coronavirus was already known about then that could be a candidate (Menachery et al., 2015, 2016).

A report produced by the National Academies of Sciences, Engineering, and Medicine; Health and Medicine Division; Board on Global Health; Committee on Global Health and the Future of the United States (2017, 15th May) outlined in some detail the future threats and risks associated with outbreaks of new pathogens for which no vaccines or effective therapeutic treatments were available. The principal threat derived from so-called zoonotic viruses that jump from one species to another. Over time, the ability of humans to protect themselves from new diseases had grown primarily through scientific discoveries and associated new medical treatments, including a range of preventative measures (i.e., vaccines) and treatment drugs. The main concern for the future was that if a new zoonotic virus jumped into humans and caused severe symptoms and even death for some (or many), there would be no pharmaceutical protections available. Many people could end up in hospitals overwhelming health services and resulting in many deaths. The only interventions available to tackle such pandemics would entail extensive closure of societies and their economies. This would be especially necessary with airborne viruses. The cures could be as damaging as the disease.

Various ongoing changes and trends caused by humans were contributing to increased risks of zoonotic virus pandemics. One principal factor was the increased urbanisation of many societies that was destroying the natural habitats of wild animals that could harbour zoonotic viruses which resulted in those animals living in closer proximity to humans. Another factor was the progressive globalisation of economies that resulted in greater movements of people and goods between countries. Both of these factors could convey viruses vary rapidly around the world. Hence, highly infectious diseases can potentially be more readily seeded and more extensively spread than at any previous time. They represent a real threat to the well-being of nations. Experts studying these diseases had been issuing warnings for many years and certainly throughout the 21st century that countries needed to be better prepared to deal with pandemics. While global pandemics occurred only occasionally, there were signs that another was overdue and that the conditions under which a major outbreak of a new virus to which humans had no natural immunity had grown in prevalence (Mackenzie, 2020).

During the 21st century alone, there were a number of outbreaks of diseases including avian influenza, Ebola, hantavirus, Marburg, MERS and SARS that occurred either through zoonotic viruses or pathogens that had infiltrated specific communities with which others then came into contact. Increased urbanisation has had the impact of decreasing the biodiversity of specific environments that have also created opportunities for these and other established diseases such as tuberculosis, to thrive and among populations with little or no in-built resistance (Pongsiri et al., 2009; Allen et al., 2010).

In 2019, Dan Coats, the Director of National Intelligence, issued a Worldwide Threat Assessment and concluded that the United States (and the rest of the world) would be vulnerable to the next flu pandemic or largescale outbreak of a contagious disease. It could cause large numbers of deaths and have serious effects on economies (Coats, 2019, 29th January).

COVID-19: First Signs

US intelligence agencies had learned in November 2019 about a new viral contagion sweeping through China's Wuhan region which had impacted upon the way businesses operated and people went about their normal lives. Early reports indicated that this new disease posed a serious threat to the population. This outbreak eventually turned out to be caused by the novel coronavirus that swept across most other parts of the world in the months ahead. It was reported that this evidence was presented to the National Security Council, the Pentagon and the White House. Further briefings were presented to key policymakers and decision-makers in the United States federal government. It was further noted that for any of these reports to be presented at this level, they would have had to go through a process of serious vetting and verification that probably would have taken weeks. It was concluded from these initial assessments that the Chinese leadership knew that the epidemic was out of control and concealed important information about it from foreign governments and international public health agencies (Margolin & Meek, 2020, 9th April).

Another report appeared in the autumn 2019 based on research undertaken by the Economist Intelligence Unit (EIU) working with the Nuclear Threat Initiative (NTI) and the Johns Hopkins Center for Health Security (CHS) that assessed the threats from and preparedness of different nations and their health systems to prevent, detect and respond to major new pandemics (McGrath, 2019, 25th October). The conclusions reached were neither positive nor reassuring. Most countries were thought to be ill-prepared for such a catastrophe. Their societies could be seriously undermined by major biological events whether triggered by the spread of a new naturally occurring pathogen or an engineered organism. A Global Health Security Index was developed with input from a group of international experts from 13 countries. Countries were scored on a 100-point scale, on which a score of 100 indicated being fully prepared. The average score was 40.2. Even amongst the 60 highest income nations, the average score was only 51.9. The UK's score was 77.9, the second highest after the United States. Yet, as the 2020 pandemic eventually demonstrated, this evaluation is probably rather flattering.

Globally, it is the responsibility of the WHO to identify new diseases and epidemics and to initiate appropriate responses in partnership with relevant national governments. The WHO reacted swiftly once it was established that a new respiratory virus had been detected in Wuhan, China, orchestrating information dissemination to health authorities around the world and producing guidelines for national health systems based on rapidly accumulating scientific and clinical understanding about it. In examining WHO-initiated actions and events over the January to April period in 2020, when the virus spread globally, it is clear that from early on, there were concerns that national governments around the world were not prepared to tackle this pandemic and many underestimated the risk it posed to their populations.

While events of this kind happen once in a lifetime at most, a mixture of complacency and ill-preparedness meant that the new virus spread rapidly through the populations of numerous countries – even those living in the most highly developed countries in the world – and quickly threatened to overwhelm even the best-resourced health services. In the United Kingdom, there was initial government inaction during a period when the WHO, was issuing severe warnings about the possible impact of this new disease and then adoption of the wrong approach in trying to reduce infection rates because of flawed psychological thinking about the kinds of interventions and restrictions people would tolerate.

By the time a harsher approach was adopted, the virus had already spread far and wide. Fortunately, most of those infected either experienced no symptoms or only mild ill effects. For an unlucky minority, however, the virus could cause serious respiratory illness requiring hospitalisation and for a few it could be deadly. Those at serious risk comprised only a tiny portion of the population in percentage terms, but when translated into numbers of cases, they reached the tens of thousands and this was enough to place the country's National Health Service under great strain, and quite possibly, according to some epidemiological modelling, overwhelming its ability to cope.

Historical Pandemics and Interventions

The COVID-19 pandemic was not the first time the world had experienced a major disease outbreak that spilled out beyond the borders of a single nation. During the Spanish flu pandemic that spread around the globe at the end of the First World War and subsequently killed tens of millions and made many more ill, many authorities reacted by shutting down specific activities and public spaces and placed responsibility of the public also to do the right thing. Schools were closed, and mass gatherings of people were banned. People that became sick were quarantined or isolated themselves to protect others. More recent coronavirus-based outbreaks (SARS-CoV-1 and MERS) had occurred in the 21st century but had been largely restricted to Asia. The countries affected by these viruses however learned valuable lessons from these outbreaks that served them well when SARS-CoV-2 broke out.

The 1918 influenza pandemic had high worldwide infection and mortality rates and triggered a number of different public health interventions on the part of national governments in an effort to contain the disease. The extent of this pandemic varied around the world. There was considerable geographic variance in the spread of the disease across the United States, for instance, compared to Europe. In many places, there were three peaks to this disease before it finally died out. In the United States, however, some cities experienced only one large peak, while others saw two.

There were a range of non-pharmaceutical interventions deployed across the United States during the Spanish Flu outbreak. Many of these resonate with similar interventions used during the 2020 SARS-CoV-2 pandemic. Many cities closed churches, dance halls, schools and theatres. In some places, weddings and funerals were restricted to 20 attendees. Some cities required their citizens to wear face masks and others did not. In general, the more far-reaching were the restrictions, the more effective they were at suppressing the spreading of the disease. The best-performing city had a peak mortality rate that was only one-eighth of that of the worst-performing city. Furthermore, in the best performer, these interventions were deployed within two days of the first cases being identified whereas the worst performer waited two weeks before acting (Hatchett et al., 2007).

Comparisons of excess mortality rates in the United States, that is death rates specifically attributable to this flu over and above normal death rates, varied from city to city and that cities that experienced an initial high peak of infection were the ones most likely to experience a second peak. Research also indicated that the implementation of interventions might offset the spread of the virus, but in most places where this happened, the impact amounted to only a 10–30% reduction in mortality. A few cities fared better than this with mortality reductions reaching 30–50%. Much depended on the timing of the interventions. If these were introduced too late or relaxed too soon, the pandemic could take hold again and mortality levels rose (Bootsma & Ferguson, 2007).

In America, the city that was eventually the most successful in controlling the spread of Spanish influenza in 1918 was St Louis, Missouri. In comparing its performance with the remainder of the nine largest cities in the country. Analysis showed that its timely introduction of public health interventions, most especially banning large public gatherings, was a critical factor. Although St Louis experienced a second wave of infection, it peaked at a far lower level than across the other major cities of the United States (Kalnins, 2006).

Non-pharmacological interventions to confront pandemic outbreaks have a mixed history of effectiveness and whether they eventually make any significant difference to the spread of an infection depends upon their nature and how and when they are implemented. Although pharmacological drug treatments may ultimately be the only way of helping someone infected and vaccines may be needed to provide longer-term protection against a new virus that has infected the human species, these protections are not usually available initially. Hence, it can often be necessary to take other steps to control rates of spread of new diseases. These tend to be social and behavioural interventions and can result in upsetting people's lives in significant ways.

Non-pharmacological interventions do not provide cures. They are simply delaying tactics designed to reduce the penetration of a disease in a population until pharmacological treatment becomes available. Further research into the impact of public health interventions to control the spread of Spanish flu in 1918 in the United States investigated the nature of specific interventions deployed across American cities and their impact in relation to excess death rates over a 26-weeks period after the virus hit. The key interventions were school closures, cancellation of public gatherings and isolation and quarantining of symptomatic cases. Not all cities implemented every one of these measures.

A number of locations implemented school closures and public events bans, while others also deployed isolating of known cases. The first two interventions used together were found to reduce excess death rates, managed to delay peak death rates and had lower peak mortality rates. The impact of these interventions was made stronger if they had been implemented earlier rather than later in the progression of the pandemic. Sustaining the interventions for longer also delivered dividends in terms of overall excess death rates (Markel et al., 2007).

Pandemics and Collateral Damage

The COVID-19 pandemic was frequently presented as a completely new and unprecedented experience for most people for those living in Western countries. In contrast, in the East, there had been regional pandemics involving coronaviruses and influenzas. This earlier and relevant experience is perhaps one of the main reasons why some countries in the Far East reacted so swiftly and firmly to get a grip on the early spread of COVID-19. While not all Far Eastern countries responded in the same ways, many already had clearly articulated plans for coping with large-scale infectious disease outbreaks and were well equipped in advance to implement them. In each case, they had a strategy that has proven to be effective for them, whether it took the form of extensive lockdowns on people's gatherings and movements or targeted testing, tracing and quarantining of the infected (Cascella et al., 2020).

Yet, it would be wrong to claim that the West had no prior pandemic experience. As noted already, 100 years earlier, the West was ravaged by the Spanish Flu pandemic. More recently, during the post-Second World War era, further influenza outbreaks that started in the East and in one case in the West provided further warnings about the risks of new viruses spreading rapidly around the world. The late 20th century outbreaks caused minimal side effects for societies, but did produce local disruptions. The Spanish Flu pandemic had more pronounced collateral damage that was felt socially and economically.

Modern medical science tackles new viruses through vaccines and drug therapies to protect humans from their worst effects. If these viruses get out of control, however, in the absence of medical interventions of proven effectiveness, governments and their public health systems must turn to other methods to keep people safe. These methods have tended to include taking symptomatic people away from the remainder of the population and placing them in isolation or quarantine so that they cannot give the disease to others, closing down physical spaces in which people are most often likely to mix in large numbers, and getting people to take personal protective steps such as wearing face masks or being more diligent about personal hygiene.

The Spanish flu outbreak in the early 20th century was generally regarded as having three waves. The first occurred in the spring 1918, then another in the autumn of the same year and then again in the winter of 1918–1919. The first and third waves were relatively mild, but the second wave caused massive losses of life. An initial calculation of the mortality rate estimated 21.5 million deaths, but this later revised up to double that figure (Johnson & Mueller, 2002; Guan et al., 2010; Humphries, 2013). Most of the deaths occurred in the second wave (Barry, 2004b).

One of the lessons learned from the Spanish flu pandemic was that it caused a great deal of collateral damage. While it did make many people ill and killed millions, it had other profound effects that mostly stemmed from the non-pharmaceutical interventions deployed to tackle the spreading of the disease and also from its physical impact on economies in terms of high levels of absenteeism at work, businesses and schools being closed down, with some even going bankrupt as a result (USDHHS, 2016). One feature of this disease, which differentiated it from the 2020 coronavirus pandemic, was that it disproportionately affected younger people and this meant that it hit the workforce especially hard (Johnson & Mueller, 2002; Humphries, 2013).

There were no vaccines available to control these viral outbreaks. During the Spanish flu outbreak, this meant that public health authorities, state and national governments had to rely on non-pharmaceutical interventions. These included quarantines, school closures, bans on public gatherings, personal hygiene practices such as covering the mouth and nose when coughing and sneezing and wearing face masks (Markel et al., 2006).

The use of these restrictions in different parts of the United States was found to reduce mortality rates from this influenza. The best strategies used a combination of restrictions rather than being reliant on just one or two. School closures and bans on public gatherings were found to be especially effective when part of the mix. The timing of restrictions also emerged as a crucial factor. It is important to impose these interventions early, that is, with days of detecting surges in case numbers and not to open up too soon. The removal of non-pharmaceutical interventions too soon could result in the virus being resurgent (Markel et al., 2006). All these lessons were learned one hundred years ago.

Further influenza pandemics occurred in 1957–1958 (Asian Flu), 1968–1970 (Hong Kong Flu) and in 2009–2010 (Swine Flu). These originated in mainland

China, Hong Kong and Mexico, respectively. Asian flu spread to surrounding Asian countries and to the United States and Eastern Europe. Hong Kong flue spread to Europe, Northern America and Australia. Swine flu spread to 122 countries within three months of being detected. Asian flu affected younger age groups the most and there was some social disruption caused by school and workplace absenteeism. The economic impact was minimal with the impact on GDP in North America calculated at around 1%. The Hong Kong flu also affected younger people the most. Some schools closed and student and employee-absenteeism rates increased for a time. Once again, the wider social and economic damage was minimal.

Swine flu had the most significant effects among children, young adults and pregnant women. It caused some social disruption and economic losses in countries most badly hit ranged between a 0.5% and 1.5% reduction in GDP. Key behavioural contributors were absenteeism from work and reduced tourism (Saunders-Hastings & Krewski, 2016). Non-pharmaceutical measures comprised campaigns for enhanced hand hygiene and the isolation of symptomatic individuals. Some countries, including Australia, the United Kingdom and the United States also considered and implemented school closures.

As well as the economic damage caused by the impact of pandemics on businesses and other employers in the form of absenteeism and mandated social isolation, these outbreaks, when they occur on a national or international scale and persist over time, can produce adverse psychological side-effects. It is these effects that are the focus of this book. Pandemics can cause significant levels of uncertainty about health risks as well as economic risks. These enhanced risk perceptions can trigger anxiety or fear responses. This reaction was observed during the 1918–1920 Spanish flu pandemic (Ott et al., 2007; Parmet & Rothstein, 2018).

The 2020 COVID-19 pandemic received wall-to-wall media coverage and dominated news agendas around the world. The same was not true of Spanish flu. This virus was already spreading around the United States where many of those who studied this pandemic believe the outbreak began in a military base, Fort Riley Kansas City. This was never unequivocally proven, but there was compelling circumstantial evidence that this is what happened (Barry, 2004a). During the First World War, much media coverage in the West was tightly censored and largely omitted coverage of this new virus. This was not true of the media in Spain which was neutral during the war and whose press openly reported on the outbreak and how it was spreading. It was this coverage that raised the international public profile of this disease and led to it being referred to as the "Spanish flu" (Soreff & Bazemore, 2008; Short et al., 2018).

In the United States, many people were in denial about the seriousness of the outbreak. There were also those who believed in conspiracy theories about the virus. The characteristics of the blame game at that time resonated with the kinds of unproven theories about the origins of COVID-19 and blame targets believed to be responsible for its contagion. Some Americans blamed immigrant groups for the disease. Others believed that the virus was transported to the United States by German U-boats to infect the population (Barry, 2004a).

Against this backdrop of explanatory narratives, there was also a powerful anxiety response. Some Americans were fearful that this virus spelled the end of the world. In some communities, people starved to death because their friends and neighbours were afraid to go near them to deliver food. There was also evidence of increased suicide rates. Chronic anxiety symptoms led to depression for some. Others vented their frustrations and their fears through destructive behaviour in a number of settings (Wasserman, 1992; Barry, 2004a, 2004b, 2006). As time allows for reflection on the collateral damage of the COVID-19 pandemic, as this book begins to do, all of these adverse psychological responses experienced during the Spanish flu outbreak, noted 100 years earlier are echoed again.

The COVID-19 Pandemic and Impact on People's Well-Being

When the novel coronavirus (SARS-CoV-2) reached around the world, man countries in the West beyond Asia were confronted with a major public health crisis unliked any current generations had experienced before. The last pandemic on the same scale had occurred 100 years earlier with an influenza virus that came be popularly labelled as "Spanish" flu even though it had not originated in Spain (Brown, 2020). Some Asian nations had experienced regional pandemics that had hit their societies hard, but the rest of the world did not share in this experience. Initially, in the United Kingdom, there was a sense among the public that this might be yet another "Asian" virus that would have at worst only mild effects on them. It seems that many in government held a similar view as there was initially a lack of urgency about planning for a major society-wide closedown. Yet, scientists familiar with the study of such incidents had sensed early on that this virus could be a major problem even for countries thousands of miles away from where it had apparently originated in China.

Once it became clear through mounting numbers of COVID-19 cases that this could rapidly escalate into a major problem and even a national crisis, most western governments with a greater sense of urgency to tackle it. Some acted more swiftly and more severely than others. Some, such as Australia and New Zealand, closed their borders to everyone, others remained open to receive people from abroad. Some countries effectively placed their entire populations under quarantine and others (such as Sweden continued to function largely as normal with a few light-touch precautions).

In the United Kingdom, the critical policy decision to move from a light-touch approach of adoption personal protection and other voluntary behavioural measures (under guidance) to mandated closures of many businesses and public spaces and requirements on people to stay at home except for essential trips out, underlined for the public the seriousness of the situation. Once this had happened, most people were forced to embrace radical changes to the way they lived their lives. Such measures were deemed essential to protect everyone as far as possible from infection. At the same time, the protective measures imposed such draconian constraints on people's behaviour that they became a source of potential harm in their own right. This collateral damage is the focus of this book. There are important questions about public compliance with behavioural restrictions and where they turned for this relevant information. These topics are discussed in separate volumes by the author.

One major public health concern that arose during the pandemic was the status of public mental health. There was evidence that some people were clearly fearful of infection. Others were made anxious by the threats posed to their livelihoods and access to social support systems by strict behaviour constraints. In some cases, deteriorating mental health resulted in increased occurrences of destructive behaviour patterns that could be both inward-directed and aimed at others. All of these impacts represented a parallel wave of public health crises occurring alongside COVID-19. Early evidence emerged that some people adjusted to their changed circumstances. Yet, there were also clear signals that lifestyle adjustments often took a form that could lay the foundations of problematic behaviour down the road. Inevitably for many people, these restrictions represented a major change to their overall quality of life.

Researchers in the COVID-19 Psychological Research Consortium (C19PRC) investigated these impacts among people in the United Kingdom in July 2020 (in the third wave of a longitudinal study). The data were collected around three to four months after the first nationwide lockdown in the United Kingdom (Butter et al., 2021). Respondents were questioned about the lifestyle changes they had experienced and about their own assessments of the extent to which their quality of life had been affected. They were originally given a list of 19 life aspects to rate in this context. These comprised: your home life, your relationships with your intimate partner, your family, your children, your friends and your work colleagues; your diet and exercise regime, taking care of your mental health and your physical health; your work role and work–life balance, and your time spent commuting; your education and personal development, and engagement in hobbies and pastimes; your socialising, your sex life and your religious or spiritual life, and your social media use.

Five lifestyle dimensions were identified from their statistical analyses which reflected partner relationships, health, family and friend relations, personal and social activities and work–life. Seven different types of changes were identified across these categories of life experience. For the greatest proportion of respondents, there was no change in the quality of life registered (68%). Other changes noted by small minorities were: better relationships (10%), worse partner relations (7%), worse in all aspects except partner relations (6%), better in all aspects except partner relations (4%), better overall (3%) and worse overall (3%). Reporting worse partner relations and saying that quality of life was worse overall were also associated with poorer mental health, including evidence of post-traumatic stress disorder and suicidal tendencies. Hence, after four months of restrictions and cautionary advice about the pandemic, most people had not yet experienced the severe quality of life changes but for one in seven people (15%), things were reported as having got worse (Butter et al., 2021).

What emerges from this research are indications that public responses to the pandemic were diverse. The pandemic posed challenges for many people. Some people were in better shape to cope with lockdown constraints than were others. Usually, these tended to be better off households with job security and plenty of conveniently located outdoor space. Even more affluent households, however, were probably not invariably immune to the strains that "house arrest" could create on relationships. For some, relationships were strengthened by spending more time together while for others the opposite was true.

Pandemics and Mental and Behavioural Health Risks

The mental health risks of COVID-19 and related interventions were noted from very early in the pandemic. Evidence emerged from China, where researchers were quick to observe and investigate psychological side-effects of the new disease outbreak in January and February 2020, before the virus had reached many other countries. One study surveyed more than 1,000 respondents and found that 70% of them recorded moderate to high-level psychological symptoms in psychological tests. Scores were elevated for obsessive compulsivity, anxiety, interpersonal sensitivity and psychoticism. Less well-educated rural workers that were divorced or widowed and aged over 50 exhibited more than average symptoms. Relatively high risks of adverse psychological reactions were also found among children and medical staff. One major conclusion of this research was that governments needed to ensure their health systems were prepared to deal with not only those that became physically ill with the new disease but also those that experienced mental health side-effects (Tian et al., 2020).

The sentiments about the importance of focusing on mental health impacts of the pandemic were echoed in the urgings of other experts to their governments to recognise that the lived experience of a pandemic could be highly stressful for some people and at least mildly anxiety provoking for many. Although in the first weeks of the pandemic in many countries, people may have hoped that the extreme measures implemented by governments to control virus transmission between people would be short-term only, the reality that eventually materialised was quite different. Persistent restrictions, especially ones that forced any people to put their regular lives on hold ran the risk of causing chronic mental ill-health conditions to become bedded down in many. This was especially likely to occur among more vulnerable groups that already suffered from physical or mental health problems. It was therefore important for these side effects to be acknowledged by governments and public health authorities and for relevant mitigating interventions to be put in place to minimise these reactions (Holmes et al., 2020).

This book will examine a range of psychological side-effects of the COVID-19 pandemic and of the non-pharmaceutical interventions used around the world to protect people from this new and highly infectious disease. When the new virus entered humans for the first time, they had little or no natural protection against it. It therefore spread rapidly. From early on, scientists became aware that the risk of serious illness from this virus, once infected, increased with age and was greater also among those with chronic underlying health conditions. Yet, the psychological effects of the pandemic cut across all socio-demographic groups as did the emotional and behavioural effects of the interventions deployed initially to bring it under control. In reviewing the overall health impact of the pandemic, the measures taken to protect people could often be as profound as the disease itself.

References

Allen, H. K., Donato, J., Wang Cloud-Hansen, H. H., Davies, J., & Handelsman, J. (2010). Call of the wild: Antibiotic resistance genes in natural environments. *Nature Reviews Microbiology*, 8(4): 251–259.

Almutairi, K. M., Al Helih, E. M., Moussa, M., Boshaiqah, A. E., Alajilan, A. S., Vinluan, J. M., & Almutairi, A. (2015). Awareness, attitudes, and practices related to coronavirus pandemic among public in Saudi Arabia. *Family and Community Health*, 38(4): 332–340.

Barry, J. M. (2004a). *The Great Influenza: The Story of the Greatest Plague in History*. New York, NY: Viking Press.

Barry, J. (2004b) The site of origin of the 1918 influenza pandemic and its public health implications. *Journal of Translational Medicine*, 2: 3. Doi: 10.1186/1479-5876-2-3

Barry, J. M. (2006). What the 1918 flu pandemic teaches us. Yesterday's lessons inform today's preparedness. *MLO Medical Lab Observer*, 38(9): 26, 28. http://www.mlo-online.com/articles/0906/0906clinical_issues.pdf

Block, P., Hoffman, M., Raabe, I. J., Dowd, J. B., Rahal, C., Kashyap, R., & Mills, M. C. (2020). Social network-based distancing strategies to flatten the COVID-19 curve in a post-lockdown world. *Nature Human Behaviour*, 4(6): 588–596.

Bootsma, M. C. J., & Ferguson, N. M. (2007). The effect of public health measures on the 1918 influenza pandemic in U. S. cities. *Proceedings of the National Academy of Science of the United States of America*, 104(18): 7588–7593.

Brilliant, L. (2006, February). My wish: Help me stop pandemics. TED Talks. Retrieved from: https://www.ted.com/talks/larry_brilliant_my_wish_help_me_stop_pandemics?language=en

Brown, M. (2020, 23rd March). Why is the 1918 influenza virus called "Spanish flu". *USA Today News*. Retrieved from: https://eu.usatoday.com/story/news/factcheck/2020/03/23/fact-check-how-did-1918-pandemic-get-name-spanish-flu/2895617001/

Butter, S., Murphy, J., Hyland, P., McBride, O., Shevlin, M., Hartman, T. K., Bennett, K., Gibson-Miller, J., Levita, L., Martinez, A. P., Mason, L., McKay, R., Stocks, T. V. A., Vallières, F., & Bentall, R. P. (2021). Modelling the complexity of pandemic-related lifestyle quality change and mental health: An analysis of a nationally representative UK general population sample. *Social Psychiatry and Psychiatric Epidemiology: The International Journal for Research in Social and Genetic Epidemiology and Mental Health Services*. Advance online publication. https://doi.org/10.1007/s00127-021-02210-w

Cascella, M., Rajnik, M., Cuomo, A., Dulebohn, S. C., & Naopli, R. D. (2020). Features, evaluation and treatment coronavirus. Retrieved from: https://www.ncbi.nlm.nih.gov/books/NBK554776/ 25th April 2020.

Coats, D. R. (2019, 29th January). Worldwide threat assessment of the US Intelligence Community. US Senate Select Committee on Intelligence. Retrieved from: https://www.dni.gov/files/ODNI/documents/2019-ATA-SFR---SSCI.pdf

Cole, J. (2020, 26th March). Coronavirus: Why changing human behaviour is the best defence in tackling the virus. *The Conversation*. Available at: https://theconversation.com/coronavirus-why-changing-human-behaviour-is-the-best-defence-in-tackling-the-virus-134500

Cook, A. R., Zhao, X., Chen, M. I. C., & Finkelstein, E. A. (2018). Public preferences for interventions to prevent emerging infectious disease threats: A discrete choice experiment. *BMJ Open*, 8(2): e017355. DOI: 10.1136/bmjopen-2017-017355.

Cowling, B. J., Zhou, Y., Ip, D. K. M., Leung, G. M., & Aiello, A. E. (2010). Face masks to prevent transmission of influenza virus: A systematic review. *Epidemiology and Infection*, 138(4): 449–456.

Gates, Bill (2015). The next outbreak? We're not ready. TED Talks 2015. Retrieved from: https://www.ted.com/talks/bill_gates_the_next_outbreak_we_re_not_ready?language=en

Guan, Y., Yikaykrishna, D., Bahl, J., Zhu, H., Wang, J., & Smith, G. J. (2010). The emergence of pandemic influenza viruses. *Protein Cell*, 1: 9–13.

Han, E., Tan, M. M. J., Turk, E., Sridhar, D., Leung, G. M., Shibuya, K., et al. (2020). Lessons learnt from easing COVID-19 restrictions: an analysis of countries and regions in Asia Pacific and Europe. *The Lancet*, 396(10261): 1525–1534.

Hatchett, R. J., Mecher, C. E., & Lipsitch, M. (2007). Public health interventions and epidemic intensity during the 1918 influenza pandemic. *Proceedings of the National Academy of Science of the United States of America*. 104(18): 7582–7587.

Heneghan, C., & Jefferson, T. (2020, 9th April). COVID=19 deaths compared with "Swine Flu". The centre for Evidence-Based Medicine, University of Oxford, Available at: https://www.cebm.net/covid-19/covid-19-deaths-compared-with-swine-flu/

Henig, R. M. (2020, 9th April). Experts warned of a pandemic decades ago. Why weren't we ready? *National Geographic*. Retrieved from: https://www.nationalgeographic.co.uk/science-and-technology/2020/04/experts-warned-of-pandemic-decades-ago-why-werent-we-ready

Holmes, E. A., O'Connor, R. C., Perry, V. H., et al. (2020). Multidisciplinary research priorities for the COVID-19 pandemic: A call for action for mental health science. *Lancet Psychiatry*, 7: 547–560. doi:10.1016/S2215-0366(20)30168-1

Humphries, M. (2013). The first world was and the origins of the 1918 influenza pandemic. *War History*, 21: 55–81.

Jeffery, K. T., & David, M. M. (2006). 1918 influenza: The mother of all pandemics. *Emerging Infectious Disease Journal*, 12(1): 15–22.

Johnson, N., & Mueller, J. (2002). Updating the accounts: Global mortality of the 1918–1920 "spanish" influenza pandemic. *Bulletin of History of Medicine*, 76: 105–115.

Kalnins, I. (2006). The Spanish influenza of 1918 in St Louis, Missouri. *Public Health Nursing*, 23(5): 479–483.

Mackenzie, D. (2020). *COVID-19: The Pandemic that Never Should Have Happened and How To Stop the Next One*. London, UK: Little, Brown.

Margolin, J., & Meek, J. G. (2020, 9th April). *Intelligence Report Warned of Coronavirus as early as November*. ABC News. Retrieved from: https://abcnews.go.com/Politics/intelligence-report-warned-coronavirus-crisis-early-november-sources/story?id=70031273

Markel, H., Lipman, H. B., Navarro, J. A., Sloan, A., Michalsen, J. R., Stern, A. M., & Cetron, M. S. (2007). Nonpharmaceutical interventions implemented by US cities during the 1918–1919 influenza pandemic. *Journal of the American Medical Association*, 298(6): 644–654.

Markel, H., Stern, A. M., Navarro, J. A., Michaelsen, J. R., Monto, A. S., & DiGiovanni, C, Jr. (2006). Nonpharmaceutical influenza mitigation strategies, US communities, 1918–1920 pandemic. *Emerging Infectious Diseases*, 12: 1961–1964.

McGrath, C (2019, 25th October). Pandemic warning: Terrifying new report warns every country on Earth is at risk. *Express*. Retrieved from: https://www.express.co.uk/news/world/1195719/global-pandemic-ebola-epidemic-pathogen-disease-biological-warfare-latest-news-update

Menachery, V. D., Yount, B. L., Jr., Debbink, K., Agnihothram, S., Gralinski, L. E., Plante, J. A., Graham, R. L., Scobey, T., Ge, X.-I., Donaldson, E. F., Randell, S. H., Lanzaecchia, A., Marasco, W. A., Shi, Z-L., & Baric, R. S. (2015). A SARS-like cluster of circulating bat coronaviruses shows potential for human emergence. *Nature Medicine*, 21: 1508–1513.

Menachery, V. D., Yount, B. L., Jr., Sims, A. C., Debbink, K., Agnihothram, S. S., Gralinski, L. E., Graham, R. L., Scobey, T., Plante, J. A., Royal, S. R., Swanstrom, J., Sheahan, T. P., Pickles, R. J., Corti, D., Randell, S. H., Lanzavecchia, A., Marasco, W. A., & Baric, R. S. (2016). SARS-like WIV1-CoV poised for human emergence. *Proceedings of the National Academy of Sciences of the United States of America*, 113(11): 3048–3053. DOI: 10.1073/pnas.1517719113

National Academies of Sciences, Engineering, and Medicine; Health and Medicine Division; Board on Global Health; Committee on Global Health and the Future of the United States. (2017, 15th May). *Global Health and the Future Role of the United States*. Washington DC: National Academies Press. Available at: https://www.ncbi.nlm.nih.gov/books/NBK458474/

Ngonghala, C. N., Iboi, E., Eikenberry, S., Scotch, M., MacIntyre, C. R., Bonds, M. H., & Gumel, A. B. (2020). Mathematical assessment of the impact of non-pharmaceutical interventions on curtailing the 2019 novel Coronavirus. *Mathematical Biosciences*, 325(108364). DOI: 10.1016/j.mbs.2020.108364

Ott, M., Shaw, S. F., Danila, R. N., & Lynfield, R. (2007). Lessons learned from the 1918-1919 influenza pandemic in Minneapolis and St. Paul, Minnesota. *Public Health Reports (Washington, D.C. 1974)*, 122(6): 803–810. 10.1177/003335490712200612

Parmet, W. E., & Rothstein, M. A. (2018). The 1918 Influenza Pandemic: Lessons learned and not-introduction to the special section. *American Journal of Public Health*, 108(11): 1435–1436. 10.2105/AJPH.2018.304695

Pongsiri, M. J., Roman, J., Ezenwa, V. O., Goldberg, T. L., Koren, H. S., Newbold, S. C., Ostfeld, R. S., Pattanayak, S. K., &. Salkeld, D. J. (2009). Biodiversity loss affects global disease ecology. *BioScience*, 59(11): 945–954.

Saunders-Hastings, P. R., & Krewski, D. (2016). Reviewing the history of pandemic influenza: Understanding patterns of emergence and transmission. *Pathogens*, 5(4): 66. 10.3390/pathogens5040066

Short, K. R., Kedzierska, K., & van de Sandt, C. E. (2018). Back to the future: Lessons learned from the 1918 influenza pandemic. *Frontiers in Cellular and Infection Microbiology*, 8: 343.

Soreff, S. M., & Bazemore, P. H. (2008, 1st February) The forgotten flu. Behavioural Health Centre Executive. Retrieved from: https://www.hmpgloballearningnetwork.com/site/behavioral/article/forgotten-flu

Tian, F., Li, H., Tian, S., et al. (2020). Psychological symptoms of ordinary Chinese citizens based on SCL-90 during the level I emergency response to COVID-19. *Psychiatry Research*, 288: 112992. doi:10.1016/j.psychres.2020.112992

USDHHS (2016). The Great Pandemic: The United States in 1918–1919. Retrieved from: http://www.flu.gov/pandemic/history/1918/index/html

Wasserman, I. M. (1992). The impact of epidemic, war, prohibition and media on suicide: United States, 1910-1920. *Suicide and Life Threatening Behaviour*, 22 (2): 240–254.

WHO (2010, August). *WHO Director-General declares H1N1 pandemic over*. Geneva, Switzerland: World Health Organization. Retrieved from: https://www.euro.who.int/en/health-topics/communicable-diseases/influenza/news/news/2010/08/who-director-general-declares-h1n1-pandemic-over

World Health Organization (2020). *Listing of WHO's Responses to COVID-19*. (Originally compiled 29th June 2020; updated on 28th December 2020). Geneva, Switzerland: World Health Organization. Retrieved from: https://www.who.int/news/item/29-06-2020-covidtimeline

Chapter 2

Lockdown Side-Effects: Public Fear

During pandemics, it is not unknown that people develop many anxiety symptoms (Ott et al., 2007; Parmet & Rothstein, 2018). They become fearful of touching potentially contaminated objects or surfaces, afraid of foreigners perceived as sources of a disease, fearful of economic circumstances of pandemic side-effects and worried about restrictions of seeing their families. They might also develop anxieties about becoming seriously ill if infected and might become obsessional about checking on the latest communications about a new disease and the steps being taken to combat it. As the opening chapter showed, these concerns characterised public reactions to the last global pandemic on the scale of COVID-19 – the Spanish flu outbreak of 2018–2020. There was evidence then that people, including some medical practitioners, were in despair that the virus could not be stopped (Schmechel et al., 2021).

Research conducted among populations infected by more recent pandemics had confirmed that the upheaval these events can cause to entire societies can give rise to severe social and psychological reactions (Arnstein et al., 2020). At the same time, the way people respond cognitively and emotionally can influence the specific coping mechanisms they adopt during a national crisis. With the first SARS (Severe Accute Respiratory Syndrome) outbreak in 2002–2003, evidence emerged that people did adopt various coping strategies. People, who tended to engage in wishful thinking, that is, imagining pleasing or positive outcomes without having compelling empirical reasons for doing so, were more likely to engage in social isolation behaviour, avoiding other people and keeping away from crowded physical spaces. Yet, these individuals were less likely to diligently follow rules about personal hygiene such as thorough and regular hand-washing and cleaning down of surfaces. Individuals, who were empathetic, were more likely to approach others even when they were at high risk of infection categories and also adopted more positive personal health behaviours (Lee-Baggley et al., 2004).

An investigation of members of the public who had come into contact with patients infected by the MERS (Middle East Respiratory Syndrome) in Korea, most (1656 out of 1692) did not catch the disease. Among the latter,

DOI: 10.4324/9781003274377-2

nearly 8% displayed symptoms of anxiety as measured by a General Anxiety Disorder psychological test. Twice as many (17%) displayed symptoms of anger (Jeong et al., 2016). A further study of American college students revealed a clear presence of swine-flu-related anxiety during the outbreak of the H1N1 virus in 2009. This took the form of general health anxiety and anxiety more acutely linked to the perceived risk of personal infection (Wheaton et al., 2012).

Early Anxiety Symptoms in the COVID-19 Pandemic

As the pandemic began to enter more and more countries and infect growing numbers of people within those countries, there was a marked initial public response of concern in a number of locations (Asmundson & Taylor, 2020). This could not be taken as evidence of a serious mental health impact of the pandemic, but it represented a foretaste of what was to come in terms of collateral damage. Even by early February 2020, one-third of Canadians said they were worried about this virus (Angus Reid Institute, 2020). Yet only four cases of COVID-19 had been recorded in the country at that point. As further evidence of public fear, there were reports of more and more people taking precautionary behaviour such as increased washing of hands (41%) and avoidance of public places (12%). Despite its generally strong reputation, one in three Canadians also started to question whether their healthcare system would be able to cope with this new disease (Angus Reid Institute, 2020).

In Canada's close neighbour, the United States, public polling at the end of January 2020, when there had been five recorded cases of people infected by the new coronavirus, more than one in three people (37%) were concerned about the virus spreading in the United States. One in four (25%) said they were more worried about this new virus than they had been about the 2014 Ebola outbreak (Morning Consult, 2020). By the beginning of February 2020, two-thirds of Americans (66%) said that this new virus was a real threat and over half (56%) were concerned about it spreading around their country (National Public Radio, 2020).

These fear responses to what become known as the "Chinese virus" also bred paranoia and xenophobia among Americans, some of which were directed towards Chinese people (Aguilera, 2020). Chinese staff were laid off from their employment and Chinese customers were banned from restaurants (Eelyn, 2020; Lowen, 2020). These extreme reactions were no doubt driven by a view growing in prevalence (32%) across the United States that China and its government were to blame for this new viral outbreak (Morning Consult, 2020).

Research in Italy, which was hit hard by the novel coronavirus before most other countries in Europe, showed that nearly one in three Italians (32%) reported high levels of anxiety, over four in ten (42%) reported high levels of distress, and over half (57%) reported poor sleep quality during the pandemic. A few (8%) even reported some degree of post-traumatic stress disorder. Those infected by COVID-19 displayed worse symptoms than did those not infected. What was apparent from this study was that as well as presenting a risk to physical health for some people, COVID-19, through the lasting fear it generated, was also a potential risk to their mental health, whether they caught the disease or not (Casagrande et al., 2020).

Data from over 20,000 Italians collected during April 2020 showed that from early on people reported psychological effects of early quarantine restrictions. Symptoms could vary from mild to moderate at this time. The study usefully indicated that these reactions could vary among different types of people. They were more severe among women than men, among the less-well educated and less well-off and among those living in larger households. These worries were greater among those whose physical health was frail and who had not been put at all during the previous week. Those living closer to areas designated as red zones, that is, where local quarantines had been implemented, exhibited more severe psychological side-effects. The findings showed, from early in the pandemic, the potential it had to cause considerable collateral damage to mental health (Bonati et al., 2021).

In Nepal, an investigation of the psychological impact of COVID-19 found that the great majority of people (89%) said they were not in distress, while just over one in ten (11%) reported experiencing moderate distress. Women, older people and those with higher educational qualifications displayed the greatest sensitivity to COVID-19 (Shrestha et al., 2020).

COVID-19 Fear among Healthcare Workers

It was not just members of the public who were fearful of COVID-19, those working in frontline public services were also made extra anxious by the pandemic (Shaukat et al., 2020). Such reactions were understandable given that those, for example, in healthcare were more exposed to infection risk than anyone else, day-in and day-out in their jobs. Nursing students in Mexico displayed similar types of fears to other people in relation to COVID-19. These included concerns about the danger of contamination, the social and economic consequences of the pandemic, xenophobia, general traumatic distress and compulsive checking about the pandemic. Higher levels of knowledge about the new disease did seem able to alleviate levels of anxiety and stress experienced (Medina Fernandez et al., 2021).

Another study of frontline nurses in Pakistan found that many were worried about the pandemic. For many this anxiety centred on their concerns about becoming infected themselves. The findings indicated that COVID-related anxiety among nurses might be sensitive to public health campaigns that aim to improve everyone's knowledge and understanding of the virus and the disease it could cause. Those participants that displayed better general health knowledge and awareness and also felt that they could exert some degree of personal control over their health tended to be less worried about COVID-19 (Mubarak, 2021).

Some public health experts reinforced the research findings that showed the calming effect of better public and professional understanding of the new coronavirus and COVID-19, the disease it caused, by advising against the use of fear in pandemic-related campaigns designed to control public behaviour. The use of fear to motivate people to accept restrictions on their movements could cause as much harm as good if overplayed (Stolow et al., 2020).

High levels of fear could encourage other negative emotions to reach the surface resulting in non-compliant behaviour or other anti-social behaviour and when persistent over time could also give rise to other adverse psychological side-effects, which will be examined further in the next chapter. During the pandemic, people could become fearful because they were worried about becoming infected themselves or worry on the same basis about their families because there were no vaccines to give advance protection against this new virus and because there was general uncertainty about how serious the entire pandemic situation was (Dhama et al., 2020; Javadi & Sajadian, 2020). The virus was spreading rapidly, daily reports told of hospitals filling with COVID patients, death figures were rising all the time, and the government adopted extreme and for most people unprecedented measures to bring the pandemic under control (Chinazzi et al., 2020).

In many countries, reports emerged from early in the pandemic that among the first deaths were those of healthcare workers (Shaukat et al., 2020). That is, doctors and nurses who worked on the frontline and whose employers had been unable to provide effective protective equipment. Unsurprisingly, then, frontline healthcare staff often experienced the highest of anxiety and stress, coupled with other psychological problems such as disrupted sleep and depression (Neto et al., 2020; Satici et al., 2020).

Dimensions of Fear

One interesting question about public fear of COVID-19 is whether it was of a similar type everywhere or whether it could vary in nature. In this context, a study of the United States set out to develop a COVID Stress Scale. The original sale contained 36 items and once completed by samples of Canadian (n = 3,479) ad US (n = 3,375) respondents revealed five different types of anxiety-inducing stressors. These comprised fears about contamination, fears about economic consequences, xenophobia, compulsive fact-checking and reassurance seeking and worry about how seriously ill they might get if infected (Taylor et al., 2020).

Researchers continued this research into a "fear of COVID-19" scale in different parts of the world (Taylor et al., 2020; Joisten et al., 2021; Taylor, 2021). A Vietnamese study found that medical students were less fearful of

COVID-19 when they were better informed in general about their health and about how to stay healthy. Hence, health literacy would seem to be important in countering any fears that the new coronavirus generated. This finding emerged in April 2020 during the early stages of the pandemic when relatively little was known about this new virus. What also emerged was that students who demonstrated greater COVID-related fear also smoke and rank more and were more likely to keep doing so during the pandemic than were those will lower levels of COVID fear (Nguyen et al., 2020).

Further research confirmed the multi-factorial nature of COVID-19 fear responses. Anxiety was triggered by concerns about becoming infected, the economic and social consequences of catching the disease, concerns about specific population sub-groups as spreaders and general stress caused by the pandemic. More anxious people were also more likely than others to self-isolate. In summary, COVID-19 was a source of anxiety and this could become compounded with prior anxieties rendering some people highly distressed by the pandemic. One of the lessons to be learned is that different types of coping mechanisms were effective among different types of people (Rachor et al., 2020).

The fear of COVID-19 scale was used among a sample in Iran and confirmed that it did provide a useful measure of people's emotional reactions to the novel coronavirus. Scores on this scale exhibited statistical links to scores on established psychological tests of anxiety and depression and also to scores on a scale designed to measure generally perceived vulnerability to disease. Heightened fear of COVID-19 was related to heightened anxiety and depression and also to stronger perceived concern about personal vulnerability to disease in general (Ahorsu et al., 2020). Researchers in India developed a similar psychological test to measure COVID-related anxiety and found that it identified two types of anxiety. One was concerned with worry about social interaction and the other was concerned worry about getting ill (Chandu et al., 2020).

YouGov polls conducted between the beginning of March and early June 2020, covering a period just before and during the first British lockdown, monitored a range of public fears stemming from the pandemic in the United Kingdom. These covered fear of infection and fears associated with the wider impact of the pandemic and of the interventions taken by the government to bring its spread under control. The key results from these various surveys are summarised in the two tables below (see: https://yougov. co.uk/topics/international/articles-reports/2020/03/17/fear-catching-covid-19).

Table 2.1 summarises the headline results concerning three different fears of getting the disease. Fear of catching the infection was measured from 1st March to 5th June 2020 and fears of becoming seriously ill or that family and friends get seriously ill were tracked from 8th May to 19th June 2020. It is worth reminding the reader that lockdown was implemented from 23rd March 2020. As this table indicates, pre-lockdown, fear of personally catching the virus was low, but climbed significantly as lockdown

Table 2.1 Public Fears of Infection of Self or Others

Fear of catching infection		Fear of becoming seriously ill		Fear that Family and friends get seriously ill	
Date	%	Date	%	Date	%
1 March	24	8 May	48	8 May	72
20 March	48	15 May	48	15 May	73
27 March	61	22 May	46	22 May	69
17 April	56	20 May	44	29 May	68
1 May	55	5 June	47	5 June	70
22 May	45	12 June	41	12 June	64
5 June	47	19 June	41	19 June	62

Source: Compiled from YouGov Coronavirus UK Polls.

Table 2.2 Public Fears of Wider Impact of Pandemic

Worry that finances will be seriously affected		Worry that they will lose their job		Worry that child's education will suffer		Fear of long-term social impact	
Date	%	Date	%	Date	%	Date	%
8 May	48	8 May	22	8 May	19	8 May	73
15 May	49	15 May	21	15 May	19	15 May	76
27 May	47	22 May	20	22 May	19	22 May	74
29 May	44	29 May	19	29 May	17	29 May	73
5 June	45	5 June	20	5 June	19	5 June	74
12 June	45	12 June	20	12 June	19	12 June	76
19 June	44	19 June	18	19 June	20	19 June	73

Source: Compiled from YouGov Coronavirus UK Polls.

approached and then climbed further in late March once lockdown had been implemented before clipping back to the immediate pre-lockdown level by early June. Fear of becoming seriously ill peaked in early May 2020 and then gradually fell away over the next month. Feats for family and friends were at a much higher level, and were fairly stable from early March to early May 2020 and then fell away by a small margin.

Table 2.2 shows that just under one in two people worried about the finances and this figure fell away slightly into mid-June. Concerns about losing a job or about their children's education being undermined were voiced by one in five or fewer people and showed little change over time. The most widespread public anxiety concerned the long-term impact of the pandemic, with over seven in ten people voicing this fear throughout May and into mid-June 2020.

A survey by Ipsos-MORI (2nd April 2020) for which fieldwork was completed between 27th and 30th March 2020 found a substantial increase in the prevalence of perceived personal threat from coronavirus with 78% registering their concern compared to 61% the week before, and before the lockdown in the United Kingdom (which started on 23rd March). A more general concern for the country was also expressed by most people (94%), an increase on the already substantial proportion of people (86%) that perceived this threat one week earlier. In fact, over six in ten people (63%) were very concerned for the country as a whole (up from 42% the week before) (Skinner, 2020, 2nd April).

Further research by Ipsos-MORI that was carried out with international samples including the British public over a month into the United Kingdom lockdown when initial conversations were being held about how to return things to some semblance of normality confirmed that many people displayed a degree of anxiety about the risks from the virus post-lockdown. A 14-country survey revealed that there was widespread public anxiety in 12 countries about the anticipated risks of leaving their homes once workplaces and public services started to open up again. This fear-of-risk sentiment was held by over seven in ten people (71%) in the United Kingdom. Similar majorities expressed this view in India (78%), Japan (77%), China (72%), Mexico (71%), Brazil (68%), Canada (68%), United States (67%), Spain (67%), Australian (64%) and France (63%). Fewer were concerned in Russia (57%), Italy (59%) and Germany (44%) (Skinner, 2020, 28th April).

This evidence from the major pollsters in the United Kingdom painted a clear picture of widespread public anxiety and fear about various outcomes of the pandemic and of their government's use of restrictions to where people could go and what they could do. As we will see, most people understood why these restrictions were in place, but nonetheless they found the uncertain future created by having their regular lives put on indefinite hold worrying. Governments had used fear to motivate behavioural compliance across their populations, presuming that relying on all people to show good sense and play along with out of a sense of civic duty and responsibility was a problematic approach that many people would be tempted to breach. By frightening everyone through an emphasis of worst-case outcomes (i.e., death) from COVID-19 and expression of infection rates that focused on numbers (that appeared large) rather than percentages of the population (that were in fact quite small), an impression was created the health risks of the new virus were greater than they really were this judgement, in turn, generated fear that would be strong enough and real enough to scare most people to comply with pandemic-related restrictions.

Public Fear about Lockdown Release

Although publics around the world eventually grew tired of lockdowns and other restrictions, for some, the relaxation of restrictions with the virus still in circulation represented another risk that also generated fear and a sense of caution (Helm et al., 2020, 3rd May). In the United Kingdom, for instance, there was evidence throughout the lockdown release period from July to September 2020 that the British people welcomed some aspects of a return to normality, but also harboured continuing fears of the risks involved in doing so.

Initially, non-essential shops reopened, along with golf courses and tennis courts, and then hairdressers, restaurants, cafes and bars. Public opinion was found to be supportive of this move because of its importance for struggling businesses. In early May 2020, as initial talk of relaxing lockdown restrictions took place, there was still a pervasive public anxiety that meant many people were not yet ready to return to normal life. People needed to be given gradual reassurances that it was safe to interact with others again under safe circumstances. The initial relaxing of lockdown measures occurred on Monday 11th May 2020 and saw rules changed on leaving home to exercise and travel as well as some leisure locations such as golf courses and garden centres being allowed to reopen. There were no longer frequency or time restrictions on exercising outdoors and more freedom was given to travel further afield outside your own area.

Measuring public opinion about these changes, YouGov found that nearly half of Britons (49%) were opposed to these changes to restrictions and significantly fewer (36%) said they were in favour of them (Ibbetson, 2020, 15th May). There were interesting differences of opinion, however, between sub-sectors of the population when defined by how they voted in the December 2019 general election. In changing the wording of questioning, YouGov asked respondents whether they thought the changes had gone too far, not far enough or were about right.

Over half of those responding (54%) believed the changes were excessive at that time, whereas nearly three in ten (29%) felt they were about right. Very few (8%) felt they did not go far enough. In a poll taken just before the new rules were introduced, YouGov found an even split (44–43%) in public support for or opposition to the changes. One of the other issues that surfaced was the clarity of public understanding about the relaxation of some lockdown restrictions. Six in ten people (60%) told YouGov that they did not understand these changes or how they would work. In spite of public caution about release from lockdown, some of the measures were welcomed. For example, eight in ten (80%) were supportive of allowing unlimited outdoor exercise. (Ibbetson, 2020, 15th May).

A survey commissioned by *The Sunday Times* revealed that many British people had not let go of cautious attitudes about coming out of lockdown, despite being frustrated by it and wanting it to end (Shipman, 2020). There seemed to be a residual fear that persisted and made many people anxious about the risks of opening up society again when the COVID-19 virus was still at large. Half of the respondents (49%), however, wanted the government to set out a plan to end the lockdown, but many others (41%) said they were still prepared to wait until they are ready to lift the lockdown. It was not clear from this survey, what was meant here by being "ready to lift the lockdown". Yet, it probably signalled that many people were still anxious about the dangers of early release of the lockdown in terms of triggering another peak in infections.

At the same time, YouGov polling in June 2020 showed that around one in five people across the United Kingdom (18–20%) feared they would lose their job. Hence, many people were conflicted in their worries. Perhaps, one indicator of just how worried they had become was signalled through the three out of four (73–76%) across June 2020 that feared the social impact of COVID-19 would be long-lasting. Public caution about coming out of lockdown was reflected in opinion about the re-opening of schools. Asked whether they would support or oppose schools being reopened in a few weeks, more people opposed (47%) than supported (28%) this idea even though there were concerns about the disruption caused to children's education (Walters, 2020, 23rd May).

It was apparent that many people preferred a staged release to the lockdown. One in four respondents told YouGov that they would like the government to release restrictions for the whole country when the time comes, many more (54%) preferred the release to occur initially in those parts of the country where the coronavirus outbreak was less severe. In the end, a prevailing and persistent fear remained among many people (48–52%) across the July to October 2020 period about catching COVID-19. Initial soundings taken after the lockdown release plan had been announced revealed that many people were fearful of returning to normal life if that might mean they were going to be placed at greater risk from COVID-19. There was also a sense that many people had grown used to being home a lot. Those working at home enjoyed the extra time it gave them to be with their families. Others had used the greater time available to them to take up old hobbies or develop new ones (Walters, 2020, 23rd May).

Public confidence in the government was not great. While many (61%) thought the government had handled things well, even more (67%) also thought it was badly prepared for the pandemic. In particular, many (62%) felt that the timing of the lockdown was too late. Opinion was evenly split between not worried (49%) and worried (48%) over the impact of the outbreak on their family finances. Looking forward and asked when they thought they would next have a foreign holiday, one in ten (10%) said later this summer (2020), one in three (33%) said next year (meaning 2021), and others (24%) thought it would be not for a couple of years or even many years. One in five (20%) felt they may never have a foreign holiday again (Walters, 2020, 23rd May).

As initial announcements were discussed about when the lockdown would be relaxed and society would begin to return to normal, in early May 2020, there was still considerable anxiety among the British public which bred caution about unlocking everything. Many people still believed it was premature to re-open schools or bars and restaurants and sports stadiums. Despite the Prime Minister's efforts to float these ideas at this time, fewer than one in five members of the public (17%) felt that the necessary conditions had been met to consider reopening schools. Many more people (67%) were opposed to this move and said they should remain closed. There was even more widespread doubt about opening up bars and restaurants again. Only one in ten (11%) felt the time was right to reopen restaurants and over three-quarters (78%) were not convinced. Fewer still (9%) would reopen pubs while over eight in ten (81%) would not. Finally, only a tiny proportion (7%) would allow mass gatherings (Helm et al., 2020).

Fear as Motivator

Fear can motivate people to change their behaviour. When and how to use fear in public health campaigns has triggered many ethical arguments. Fear can generate unpleasant feelings in people. Yet, if it encourages them to change their behaviour in ways that will protect their well-being, especially in times of national crisis, then these negative side-effects might be seen as justified (Fairchild & Bayer, 2021).

Fear had been found to work in previous public health campaigns. With fear, however, there is a downside. If it persists for a while, it can become embedded in the psyche to a degree whereby it is difficult to let go. Even when behavioural restrictions are relaxed, many people may remain fearful of recapturing their freedoms once again.

Even when using fear appeals, it remains important to feed people factual details as well so that they understand the reasons for using fear. If the founding arguments of a health campaign are unsound, fear can produce unwanted or unhelpful outcomes (Simpson, 2017). Hence, the use of fear should have evidential support in terms of its relevance to a campaign. It should be appropriate in magnitude to drive desired behaviour. There should be outcomes are result from this motivation that eventually relieve the fear so that it does not persist and become debilitating (Soames Job, 1988). This approach is also likely to receive more ethical plaudits. In the longer term, facts will also prove to be more effective than fear in maintaining safe behavioural protocols (Pomeroy, 2020). By doing this, the public will be better equipped to recognise and question the large amount of factually incorrect or fake news and ill-informed conspiracy theories in circulation about COVID-19.

Lockdown and General Mood States

Pollsters that tracked national mood states over time and analytics that track the use of specific search terms on major Internet search engines, such as Google, can provide insights into the public's emotional state. Research started to emerge that the pandemic and lockdown had measurable effects on the public's mood. Analysis of data from YouGov's mood tracker from June 2019 to June 2020 revealed that the early pandemic had a strong and generally negative effect on the British public's mood. This poll measured public mood states using 12 descriptors: happiness, contentment, inspiration, optimism, energy levels, sadness, apathy, stress, boredom, frustration, loneliness and fear (Fabian et al., 2020).

As the pandemic began to bite within the United Kingdom, negative mood states showed a progressive upturn. After the early stages of lockdown, however, these mood shifts returned back to more normal levels. There were variations in how people reacted, however, and while some moods improved others got worse. After lockdown had been implemented, apathy, boredom, frustration and loneliness levels increased. Yet, so too did feelings of contentment, happiness, inspiration and optimism. At the same time, feelings of fear, sadness and stress fell once lockdown had started. A more general perception of life satisfaction took a dive as the pandemic took hold, but then improved during lockdown (Fabian et al., 2020).

When Google Trends data were examined based on the volumes worldwide of the use of specific search terms, such as "apathy", "boredom", "fear", "psychological stress" and "sadness", the polling data patterns were reinforced. Negative affect trends found in web searches mirrored those observed in weekly mood polling trackers. Negative mood states became more prevalent in their presence in online searches as the pandemic grew, and then fell away after lockdown. This was true not just for the United Kingdom, but also for other countries such as Australia, Canada, India, Ireland, New Zealand, South Africa and the United States (Fabian et al., 2020).

The rise in negative mood states as the pandemic took hold was no doubt motivated by the increased uncertainty created by this event in terms of personal health and safety, the economic impact of lockdown actions, and the prospect of social isolation and not being able to see family members and friends. For those used to commuting, however, home-working might have restored healthier work-life balance by enabling more contact with immediate family members if you all lived under the same roof. For women, the extra strain caused by having to spend more time looking after their children when schools closed together with the responsibility for home-schooling could have caused additional anxiety. At the same time, for some women being at home all the time with their partner could give rise to greater tension leading to domestic arguments and even violence.

Evidence emerged that lockdown affected individuals living alone more than those living with someone. Those living alone were effectively cut off from their social contacts by rules prohibiting people from different households from intermingling socially. Women were more affected in a negative way than were men by the pandemic and during the early stages of lockdown. As lockdown wore on, however, their mood state improved. There was further evidence that the pandemic and initial lockdown affected the mood states of those who worked casually or part-time rather than those in full-time and well-established jobs. The former were accustomed to living off small incomes and with benefits made available during the lockdown were still able to live life much as normal, in terms of disposable income. For those experiencing larger income drops, their overall mood state was badly affected. Those on large and protected incomes had a different experience and found that they were able to save a lot of their income because there were few things still available to spend it on (Fabian et al., 2020).

Overall, the pandemic and lockdown did influence the subjective well-being of many people. Governments could help to alleviate this impact by reducing the stress caused by the pandemic and much of this stemmed from economic uncertainties. Therefore, the provision of financial support in the short-term to ensure everyone had enough income to survive and buy essentials was extremely important. In the longer-term, as the lockdown was released, further government support might be needed for employers struggling to keep going after enforced closure for many months.

YouGov's Mood Tracker, as we have just seen, monitored public mood states across the United Kingdom for long before the pandemic. Further analysis of these data spanning 2019 and 2020 has been published elsewhere. This tracker revealed that the British public's mood had displayed volatility across 2019 and especially around the end of the year when a General Election was held. During the week of the election, YouGov detected an increase in the proportion of people saying they felt "sad" (33%), an increase on the week before (26%). Across the same period, there was also an increase in the percentages of people saying they felt "scared" (up from 11% to 17%) (Smith, 2020, 2 July).

After the election, both of these figures returned to their pre-election lower levels. These responses therefore probably reflected a growth in feelings of uncertainty among the electorate about the election outcome and what kind of government the country could end up with. Clearly, the eventual outcome appeared to uplift more people than it depressed. Of course, this pattern was not universal and not surprisingly reflected a partisan divide. Labour supporters were more inclined to feel "sad" after the election than before it (38% versus 24%), presumably seeing little to celebrate in the Conservative Party's resounding election victory (Smith, 2020, 2nd July).

YouGov found a temporary Christmas boost to the public mood, with more people saying they felt "happy" during Christmas week (61%) than during the week before (48%). The cheer of the holidays soon dissipated in January as everyone returned to work and normal life again. It was during this period when the first media coverage emerged about a new virus that appeared to cause pneumonia-like symptoms among people in central China. At that time, few people in the United Kingdom thought this would be a problem for them. Over the next two months, all this changed and along with it there was a shift in the public mood. During early March, between the 6th and 23rd of the month "happiness" dropped from 50% to 25%, "optimism" fell from 24% to 16% and "contentment" fell from 29% to 13%. Feeling "scared" increased from 13% to 6% and feeling "stressed" also rose from 42% to 50%. At the point at which the lockdown was fully implemented on 23rd March 2020, one in five people (19%) said they were "bored", and one week later, this figure had increased to one in three (34%) (Smith, 2020, 2nd July).

All these negative mood shifts were temporary, however. Boredom peaked by mid-May at 40%, but by the end of June, it had already fallen to 31%. This was still well above the pre-lockdown level (19%), but indicated that either people were getting used to doing very little or had found ways of adapting to their changed circumstances to amuse themselves. Fear feelings continued to remain at the initial lockdown but showed some slight downward trending by June 2020. There was some evidence also that parts of the population felt lonely (19% at the start of lockdown). Loneliness was expected to be an issue for those most at risk of dying from COVID-19 who were required to "shield" for indefinite periods. Overall, though, loneliness claims hardly changed from pre-lockdown levels (17%) (Smith, 2020, 2nd July).

Deirdre Barrett, a psychologist at Harvard Medical School, collected accounts of more than 6,000 dreams linked to COVID-19 from around 2,400 people. Lockdown experienced characterised many people's dreams including themes of loneliness, isolation through anxiety to imagining becoming ill or overrun by pestilence (Ore, 2020). A YouGov poll in the US conducted at the beginning of April in the earliest phase of the lockdown found that 7% could recall having dreamt with the last month. Among young people aged 18–34, 9% reported having had a COVID-19-related dream. People aged 55+ (5%) were less likely to report COVID-19 dreams (Bulkeley, 2020).

Pandemic Anxiety, Stress and Adaptation

As the evidence reviewed in this chapter has shown, publics around the world were rendered in a state of fear and anxiety. For some people, these psychological responses were relatively short-lived as they developed coping mechanisms after overcoming the initial shock and surprise of their society being "locked down" and being told by their government not to leave home. Such draconian instructions were unprecedented for most people and turned their lives upside down. Feeling more anxious was to be expected.

Daily government briefings and media news report that focused on death rates from COVID-19 triggered understandable fear in people. As opinion polls showed, these fears varied with different consequences, and different fears demonstrated varied in prevalence and resilience. What became a matter of greater concern, especially for public health authorities as well as sufferers themselves, was that for some individuals, initial fear responses that are normally associated with threatening environmental conditions (and are usually temporary), turned into more chronic psychological states that persisted and could be debilitating. Such chronic psychological states often sprang from the social deprivation forced upon many people by strict social distancing rules. Anxiety and depression can often flow from or be catalysed by loneliness and being deprived of sufficient physical contact with those upon whom we most rely as sources of social and psychological sustenance. The next chapter moves forward from the psychological responses noted here to consider the scale and severity of more permanent and adverse psychological effects of the pandemic.

As an appetiser to what is to follow, a review of 21 relevant studies from different countries showed that around one in five people (out of a total of more than 82,000 studied by these investigations) reported mental health effects of COVID-19 quarantine. These effects were manifest most usually in the form of higher overall psychological distress, signs of depression and PTSD symptoms (Cavicchioli et al., 2021).

Not everyone reacted emotionally in the same way to the pandemic and to governments' interventions to bring the spreading of the new coronavirus under control via behavioural restrictions. An online survey of over 2,000 Americans conducted during March 2020 again found that women and older people exhibited more psychological distress than others in response to the pandemic. Those who had pre-existing physical health concerns, mental illness, and who were Hispanic Americans were also more likely than most to experience more severe psychological reactions to the pandemic (French et al., 2020).

The fact that COVID stress might get mixed up with other psychological problems and be magnified by them meant that it was important to differentiate between different potential causes of psychological distress in order to tease out the specific effects of the pandemic. For some people, the COVID-related behavioural restrictions were disturbing and the magnitude of this effect could be quantified. In other cases, anxiety responses were triggered to an uncertain extent by pre-existing mental health problems. Differentiating between these causes was important from the perspective of identifying and implementing relevant interventions in enabling individuals to cope with their distress more effectively (Taylor, 2021).

Further evidence emerged that public perceptions of the new coronavirus and the risks associated with it fed into more emotional responses, but that, over time, in many people initial signs of distress gradually lessened. Hence, people with stronger concerns about death from COVID-19, concerns also about the financial risks of government and public health restrictions, and those who may have lost their jobs or experienced lifestyle changes they had not chosen for themselves also displayed the greatest psychological distress in the early phase of the pandemic across March and April 2020. By June, however, further soundings revealed some lessening of distress. It also appeared from the data that as perceived risks change, anxiety levels followed suit (Robinson & Daly, 2021).

In the next few chapters, further attention is turned to adverse psychological side-effects of the pandemic that include people's reactions to the virus and to governments' and public health authorities' interventions designed to slow rates of virus transmission. The psychological effects on adults and children are examined separately although they often have symptoms in common. Evidence has been presented in this chapter that people in different parts of the world exhibited fear responses when first confronted with COVID-19 and that these responses persisted over many months. One of the great concerns about these responses has been whether they convert into longer-term and potentially debilitating psychological ill-health outcomes. It is also important to understand whether there have been specific mechanisms through which these persistent and chronic mental health conditions become established. One of these is the social isolation that characterised the dominant suite of interventions based on physical distancing. One immediate psychological response to isolation is a feeling of loneliness and if this feeling persists over time, it can create the psychological conditions that promote mental health problems. This is the topic of the next chapter.

References

Aguilera J. Time (2020). Xenophobia "is a pre-existing condition." how harmful stereotypes and racism are spreading around the coronavirus. https://time.com/5775716/xenophobia-racism-stereotypes-coronavirus/

Ahorsu, D. K., Lin, C. Y., Imani, V., Saffari, M., Griffiths, M. D., & Pakpour, A. H. (2020). The fear of COVID-19 scale: Development and initial validation. *International Journal of Mental Health and Addiction*, 27: 1–9. doi: 10.1007/s11469-020-00270-8. Epub ahead of print.

Angus Reid Institute (2020). Half of Canadians taking extra precautions as coronavirus continues to spread around the globe. http://angusreid.org/wp-content/uploads/2020/02/2020.02.04_Coronavirus.pdf Retrieved February 6, 2020.

Arnstein, A., Alfani, G., Gandolfi, F., & Le Moglie, M. (2020, 22nd March). Pandemics and social capital: From Spanish flu 1918-19 to COVID-19. VOXEU/CEPR. Retrieved from: https://voxeu.org/article/pandemics-and-social-capital

Asmundson, G. J. G., & Taylor, S. (2020). Coronaphobia: Fear and the 2019-nCoV outbreak. *Journal of Anxiety Disorders*, 70: 102196. doi: 10.1016/j.janxdis.2020.102196

Awad, E., Kim, R., Schulz, J., Henrich, J., Shariff, A., Bonnefon, J.-F., & Rahwan, I. (2018). The Moral Machine experiment. *Nature*, 563: 59–64.

Beaver, K., Pedley, K., & Garrett, G. (2020, 18th November). Young Britons most likely to break coronavirus rules in the pursuit of romance. *Ipsos MORI*. Retrieved from: https://www.ipsos.com/ipsos-mori/en-uk/young-britons-most-likely-break-coronavirus-rules-pursuit-romance-0

Bonati, M., Campi, R., Zanetti, M., Cartabia, M., Scarpellini, F., Clavenna, A., & Segre G. (2021). Psychological distress among Italians during the 2019 coronavirus disease (COVID-19) quarantine. *BMC Psychiatry*, 21(1): 20. doi: 10.1186/s12888-020-03027-8

Briñol, P., & Petty, R. E. (2009). Source factors in persuasion: A self-validation approach. *European Review of Social Psychology*, 20: 49–96.

Bulkeley, K. (2020, 12th April). Common themes in dreams about the pandemic. Psychology Today. Retrieved from: https://www.psychologytoday.com/gb/blog/dreaming-in-the-digital-age/202004/common-themes-in-dreams-about-the-pandemic

Casagrande, M., Favieri, F., Tambelli, R., & Forte G. (2020). The enemy who sealed the world: Effects quarantine due to the COVID-19 on sleep quality, anxiety, and psychological distress in the Italian population. *Sleep Medicine*, 75: 12–20. doi: 10.1016/j.sleep.2020.05.011

Cavicchioli, M., Ferrucci, R., Guidetti, M., Canevini, M. P., Pravettoni, G., & Galli, F. (2021). What will be the impact of the Covid-19 quarantine on psychological distress? Considerations based on a systematic review of pandemic outbreaks. *Healthcare*, 9(1): 101. doi: 10.3390/healthcare9010101

Chandu, V. C., Pachava, S., Vadapalli, V., & Marella Y. (2020). Development and initial validation of the COVID-19 anxiety scale. *Indian Journal of Public Health*, 64(Supplement): S201–S204. doi: 10.4103/ijph.IJPH_492_20

Chinazzi, M., Davis, J. T., Ajelli, M., et al. (2020). The effect of travel restrictions on the spread of the 2019 novel coronavirus (COVID-19) outbreak. *Science*, 368: 395–400.

Dhama, K., Sharun, K., Tiwari, R., Dadar, M., Malik, Y. S., Singh, K. P., & Chaicumpa, W. (2020). COVID-19, an emerging coronavirus infection: advances and prospects in designing and developing vaccines, immunotherapeutics, and therapeutics. *Human Vaccines & Immunotherapeutics*, 16: 1232–1238

Easton, M. (2020, 20th October). *Coronavirus: How are People Breaking the Rules?* BBC News. Retrieved from: https://www.bbc.co.uk/news/uk-54620808

Evelyn K. (2020). Coronavirus: Royal Caribbean bans all Chinese nationals from its cruise ships. *The Guardian*. https://www.theguardian.com/world/2020/feb/07/coronavirus-royal-caribbean-cruise-bans-chinese-nationals Retrieved February 8, 2020.

Fabian, M., Foa, R., & Gilbert, S. (2020, 30th July). Wellbeing levels fell during the pandemic but improved under lockdown, data analysis shows. *The Conversation*. Available at: https://theconversation.com/wellbeing-levels-fell-during-the-pandemic-but-improved-under-lockdown-data-analysis-shows-143367#:~:text=Lockdowns%20are%20seemingly%20vital%20for,big%20effect%20on%20preventing%20deaths.&text=Following%20a%20rise%20in%20negative,consistently%20for%20all%20social%20groups

Fairchild, A. L., & Bayer, R. (2021, 28th January). Why using fear to promote COVID-19 vaccination and mask wearing could backfire. *The Conversation.* Retrieved from: https://theconversation.com/why-using-fear-to-promote-covid-19-vaccination-and-mask-wearing-could-backfire-153865

Freeman, A., Schneider, C. R., Dryhusrt, S., Kerr, J., Recchia, G., van der Bles, A. M., & van der Linden, S. (2020). Risk perception of COVID-19/coronavirus. Retrieved from: https://osf.io/jnu74/ 5th May 2020.

French M. T., Mortensen K., Timming A. R. (2020). Psychological distress and coronavirus fears during the initial phase of the COVID-19 pandemic in the United States. *The Journal of Mental Health Policy and Economics,* 23(3): 93–100.

Goodwin, G. P., & Landy, J. F. (2014). Valuing different human lives. *Journal of Experimental Psychology: General,* 143: 778–803.

Helm, T., McKie, R., & Jenkins, L. (2020, 3rd May). Fearful Britons remain strongly opposed to lifting coronavirus lockdown. *The Guardian.* Available at: https://www.theguardian.com/world/2020/may/02/fearful-britons-oppose-lifting-lockdown-schools-pubs-restaurants-opinium-poll

Ibbetson, C. (2020, 15th May). What do voters make of the new lockdown measures. *YouGov.* Retrieved from: https://yougov.co.uk/topics/politics/articles-reports/2020/05/15/what-do-voters-make-new-lockdown-measures

Javadi, S. M. H., & Sajadian, M. (2020). Coronavirus pandemic a factor in delayed mourning in survivors: A letter to the editor. *Journal of Arak University of Medical Sciences (JAMS),* 23: 2–7.

Jeong, H., Yim, H. W., Song, Y. J., Ki, M., Min, J. A., Cho, J., & Chae, J. H. (2016). Mental health status of people isolated due to Middle East Respiratory Syndrome. *Epidemiology and health Epidemiology and Health,* 38: e2016048.

Joisten, C., Kossow, A., Book, J., Broichhaus, L., Daum, M., Eisenburger, N., Fabrice, A., Feddern, S., Gehlhar, A., Graf, A. C., Grüne, B., Lorbacher, M., Nießen, J., Noethig, W., Schmidt, N., Tappiser, M., & Wiesmüller, G. A. (2021). How to manage quarantine-adherence, psychosocial consequences, coping strategies and lifestyle of patients with COVID-19 and their confirmed contacts: study protocol of the CoCo-Fakt surveillance study, Cologne, Germany. *BMJ Open,* 11(4): e048001. doi: 10.1136/bmjopen-2020-048001

King's College London (2020, 16th August). How the UK would be prepared to live if a Covid vaccine can't be found. Available at: https://www.kcl.ac.uk/news/how-the-uk-would-be-prepared-to-live-if-covid-vaccine-cant-be-found

Lee-Baggley, D., DeLongis, A., Voorhoeave, P., & Greenglass, E. (2004). *Asian Journal of Social Psychology,* 7(1), Special Issue: Special issue on psychology of severe acute respiratory syndrome (SARS). pp. 9–23. Publisher: Blackwell Publishing;

Lowen M. BBC News (2020). Coronavirus: Chinese targeted as Italians panic. https://www.bbc.com/news/world-europe-51370822 retrieved February 8, 2020.

Medina Fernández, I. A., Carreño Moreno, S., Chaparro Díaz, L., Gallegos-Torres, R. M., Medina Fernández, J. A., & Hernández Martínez, E. K. (2001). Fear, Stress, and Knowledge regarding COVID-19 in Nursing Students and Recent Graduates in Mexico. *Investigacion y Educacion en Enfermeria,* 39(1): e05. doi: 10.17533/udea.iee.v39n1e05

Morning Consult (2020). National tracking poll #200164. https://morningconsult. com/wp-content/uploads/2020/01/200164_crosstabs_CORONAVIRUS_Adults_ v1.pdf Retrieved February 6, 2020.

Mubarak, N., Safdar, S., Faiz, S., Khan, J., & Jaafar M. (2021). Impact of public health education on undue fear of COVID-19 among nurses: The mediating role of psychological capital. *International Journal of Mental Health Nursing*, 0(2): 544–552. doi: 10.1111/inm.12819

Natasha, S., Mansoor, A. D., & Junaid, R. (2020). Physical and mental health impacts of COVID-19 on healthcare workers: A scoping review. *International Journal of Emergency Medicine (Online)*, 13(1): 40.

National Public Radio (2020). Poll: Most Americans say U.S. "doing enough" to prevent coronavirus spread. Retrieved from: https://www.npr.org/sections/health-shots/2020/02/04/802387025/poll-most-americans-say-u-s-doing-enough-to-prevent-coronavirus-spread

Neto, M. L. R., Almeida, H. G., Esmeraldo, J. D., Nobre, C. B., Pinheiro, W. R., de Oliveira, C. R. T., Sousa, I. D. C., Lima, O. M. M. L., Lima, N. N. R., Moreira, M. M., Lima, C. K. T., Júnior, J. G., & da Silva, C. G. L. (2020). When health professionals look death in the eye: The mental health of professionals who deal daily with the 2019 coronavirus outbreak. *Psychiatry Research*, 288: 112972.

Nguyen, H. T., Do, B. N., Pham, K. M., Kim, G. B., Dam, H. T. B., Nguyen, T. T., Nguyen, T. T. P., Nguyen, Y. H., Sørensen, K., Pleasant, A., & Duong, T. V. (2020). Fear of COVID-19 Scale: Associations of its scores with health literacy and health-related behaviours among medical students. *International Journal of Environmental Research and Public Health*, 17(11): 4164. doi: 10.3390/ijerph1 7114164

Office for National Statistics (2020, 27th November). Coronavirus and the social impacts on Great Britain: 20 November 2020. Retrieved from: https://www.ons. gov.uk/releases/coronavirusandthesocialimpactsongreatbritain20november2020

O'Keefe, D. J. (2016). *Persuasion: Theory and Research*. Thousand Oaks, CA: Sage.

Opinium (2020, 21st April). Public opinion on coronavirus – 21st April. Retrieved from: https://www.opinium.co.uk/public-opinion-on-coronavirus-21st-april/ 4th May 2020.

Osborne, S. (2020, 30th June). Coronavirus: British public increasingly worried about lockdown easing, survey finds. *The Independent*. Retrieved from: https:// www.independent.co.uk/news/uk/home-news/coronavirus-lockdown-easing-pubs-restaurants-hairdressers-yougov-a9593996.html

Ott, M., Shaw, S. F., Danila, R. N., & Lynfield, R. (2007). Lessons learned from the 1918–1919 influenza pandemic in Minneapolis and St. Paul, Minnesota. *Public health reports (Washington, D.C. 1974)*, 122(6): 803–810. 10.1177/0033354 90712200612

Owen, G. (2020, 27th September). More voters fear pandemic's threat to economy than risk to their health. *Mail on Sunday*, 16–17.

Page, B. (2020, 11th October). Majority of Britons support local lockdowns, even if it impacts them directly. Ipsos-MORI. Retrieved from: https://www.ipsos.com/ ipsos-mori/en-uk/majority-britons-support-local-coronavirus-lockdowns-even-if-it-impacts-them-directly

Page, B. (2020, 20th October). Britons increasingly abiding by the COVID-19 rules, with social responsibility and the NHS the primary drivers. Ipsos-MORI. Retrieved from: https://www.ipsos.com/ipsos-mori/en-uk/britons-increasingly-abiding-covid-19-rules-social-responsibility-and-nhs-primary-drivers

Parmet, W. E., & Rothstein, M. A. (2018). The 1918 Influenza Pandemic: Lessons learned and not-introduction to the special section. *American Journal of Public Health*, 108(11): 1435–1436. 10.2105/AJPH.2018.304695

Petty, R. E., & Cacioppo, J. T. (1986). The elaboration likelihood model of persuasion. *Advances in Experimental Social Psychology*, 19: 123–205.

Pomeroy, R. (2020, 3rd March). Facts, not fear, will stop COVID-19 – so how should we talk about it? *The European Sting*, Retrieved from: https://europeansting.com/2020/03/04/facts-not-fear-will-stop-covid-19-so-how-should-we-talk-about-it/

Rachor, G. S., McKay, D., & Taylor, S. (2020). Do pre-existing anxiety-related and mood disorders differentially impact COVID-19 stress responses and coping? *Journal of Anxiety Disorders*, 74: 102271. doi: 10.1016/j.janxdis.2020.102271

Recchia, G. (2020, 21st April). Coronavirus: New survey suggests UK public supports a long lockdown. *The Conversation* Retrieved from: https://theconversation.com/coronavirus-new-survey-suggests-uk-public-supports-a-long-lockdown-136767 5th May 2020.

Robinson, E., & Daly, M. (2021). Explaining the rise and fall of psychological distress during the COVID-19 crisis in the United States: Longitudinal evidence from the Understanding America Study. *British Journal of Health Psychology*, 26(2): 570–587. doi: 10.1111/bjhp.12493

Satici, B., Gocet-Tekin, E., Deniz, M. E., & Satici, S. A. (2020). Adaptation of the Fear of COVID-19 Scale: Its association with psychological distress and life satisfaction in Turkey. *International Journal of Mental Health and Addiction*, 1 10.1007/s11469-<020-00294-0

Schmechel, C., Joensson, L., Stinnissen, S., & Walker, S. (2021). The covid-19 pandemic one year on: Parallels and lessons from Spanish flu. *The BMJ Opinion*. Retrieved from: https://blogs.bmj.com/bmj/2021/03/11/the-covid-19-pandemic-one-year-on-parallels-and-lessons-from-spanish-flu/

Shaukat, N., Ali, D. M., & Razzak, J. (2020). Physical and mental health impacts of COVID-19 on healthcare workers: a scoping review. *International Journal of Emergency Medicine*, 13, 40. https://doi.org/10.1186/s12245-020-00299-5

Shipman, T. (2020, 3rd May). Our future begins to take shape: a marathon game of whack-a-mole. *The Sunday Times*, 9.

Shrestha, D. B., Thapa, B. B., Katuwal, N., Shrestha, B., Pant, C., Basnet, B., Mandal, P., Gurung, A., Agrawal, A., & Rouniyar, R. (2020). Psychological distress in Nepalese residents during COVID-19 pandemic: A community level survey. *BMC Psychiatry*, 20(1): 491. doi: 10.1186/s12888-020-02904-6

Simpson, T. K. (2017). Appeal to fear in health care: Appropriate or inappropriate? *Chiropractic & Manual Therapies*, 25: 27. doi: 10.1186/s12998-017-0157-8

Skinner G. (2020, 8th April). Government message cutting through on COVID-19. Ipsos-MORI. Retrieved from: https://www.ipsos.com/ipsos-mori/en-uk/government-message-cutting-through-covid-19. 9th April 2020.

Skinner, G. (2020, 22nd April). Half of Britons think the government is unlikely to have a coronavirus lockdown exit strategy. Ipsos-MORI. Retrieved from: https://www.ipsos.com/ipsos-mori/en-uk/half-britons-think-government-unlikely-have-coronavirus-lockdown-exit-strategy 29th April 2020.

Skinner, G. (2020, 28th April). Britons least likely to believe the economy and businesses should open if coronavirus not fully contained. Ipsos-MORI. Retrieved from: https://www.ipsos.com/ipsos-mori/en-uk/britons-least-likely-believe-economy-and-businesses-should-open-if-coronavirus-not-fully-contained 8th May 2020.

Smith, M. (2020, 24th June). Loosening lockdown: The public view. *YouGov*. Retrieved from: https://yougov.co.uk/topics/politics/articles-reports/2020/06/24/loosening-lockdown-public-view

Smith, M. (2020, 2nd July). An emotional year: YouGov's British mood tracker. Retrieved from: https://yougov.co.uk/topics/relationships/articles-reports/2020/07/02/emotional-year-yougo

Smyth, C. (2020, 13th October). Voters back virus rules despite hit to finances. *The Times*, 8.

Soames Job, R. F. (1988). Effective and ineffective use of fear in health promotion campaigns. *American Journal of Public Health*, 78(2): 163–167. 10.2105/ajph.78.2.163

Stolow, J. A., Moses, L. M., Lederer, A. M., & Carter, R. (2020). How fear appeal approaches in COVID-19 health communication may be harming the global community. *Health Education & Behavior*, 47: 531–535.

Taylor, L. (2020, 15th July). Eight in ten Brits in favour of local lockdowns to tackle coronavirus. Kantar. Available at: www.kantar.com/inspiration/politics/eight-in-ten-in-favour-of-local-lockdowns-to-tackle-coronavirus

Taylor, S. (2021). COVID stress syndrome: Clinical and nosological considerations. *Current Psychiatry Reports*, 23(4): 19. doi: 10.1007/s11920-021-01226-y

Taylor, S., Landry, C. A., Paluszek, M. M., Fergus, T. A., McKay, D., & Asmundson, G. J. G. (2020). Development and initial validation of the COVID Stress Scales. *Journal of Anxiety Disorders*, 72: 102232. doi:10.1016/j.janxdis.2020.102232

Wace, C. (2020, 13th October). We're being made scapegoats, say Liverpool's pubs. *The Times*, pp. 8–9.

Walter, S. (2020, 24th October). Proof UK is sick of lockdown. *Daily Mail*, pp. 8–9.

Walters, S. (2020, 23rd May). Britons shun back to work plea. *Mail on Sunday*, pp. 4–5.

Wheaton, M. G., Abramowitz, J. S., Berman, N. C., Fabricant, L. E., & Olatunji, B. O. (2012). Psychological predictors of anxiety in response to the H1N1 (swine flu) pandemic. *Cognitive Therapy and Research*, 36(3): 210–218.

Chapter 3

Lockdown and Loneliness

Social contact and companionship are fundamental human needs. Even during normal times, we need to be in touch with others. This need becomes even more acute during times of great stress and distress. When social contact is taken away from us, there can be serious psychological and physical consequences. We cease to function effectively. We can become withdrawn into ourselves. Our mental state deteriorates. Ultimately, our physical health can suffer as well (McAndrew, 2016).

Any kind of profound sensory deprivation can result in a significant mental breakdown within days. Within hours we may begin to experience strange sensations. In social deprivation conditions, we might still be able to see, hear, smell, taste and feel the world around us, but where that world is severely constrained in terms of what we are allowed to do and with whom, our psychological functioning can still go away.

The Psychology of Loneliness

Long before the pandemic, psychologists were well aware of the health risks of loneliness. It is a mental state that can be extremely damaging if it persists. The COVID-19 outbreak created conditions under which everyday life was suspended by the government and this meant that many people were forcibly starved for direct, face-to-face social contact. Making people socially isolated does not harm all – for there are some with the ability to cope – but it can harm substantial numbers. In consequence, some people adopt unhealthy behaviours as coping mechanisms such as consuming more alcohol or eating more and putting on weight (Brooks et al., 2020; Holt-Lunstad et al., 2015; Hawkley and and Cacioppo, 2010). Loneliness can also have cognitive side-effects and chronic isolation has been linked to the onset of dementia (Lara et al., 2019).

Being separated from all or even most social companionship can trigger feelings of loneliness can result in harmful mental and physical health side-effects. These side-effects can be experienced within a short space of time. If they are only temporary no lasting harm may be done. If they persist,

DOI: 10.4324/9781003274377-3

however, and if the conditions triggering them are re-introduced over and over, they can result in longer-term damage (Willeumier, 2021).

Why does this happen? Social isolation, it seems, can affect brain chemistry. Experiments in which some participants were placed into social isolation settings for a limited period (e.g., 10 hours) and in some instances also showed images of people they knew enjoying themselves, functional magnetic imaging scans showed that parts of their brains became activated that are normally linked to responses to rewarding experiences and cravings. It was not simply the social isolation experience but this combined with reminders that people on the outside were enjoying experiences that the individual in the experiment was missing out on, that made the difference. The responses of people in the social isolation condition resembled those of others placed in a food deprivation condition (Tomova et al., 2020).

Loneliness: Objective or Subjective?

A major review and meta-analysis of research findings published from 1950 to 2016 concluded that social isolation was regularly found to be linked significantly to loneliness. Not only that, but loneliness could often result in a deterioration in mental health and ultimately pushed up mortality rates. Whether loneliness that stems from social isolation also increases individuals' risks of succumbing to other diseases such as cancer and cardiovascular problems was less clear. The authors of this analysis proposed, however, that this was a question worthy of further enquiry (Leigh-Hunt et al., 2017).

Further American evidence corroborated these findings among older adults aged 55 and over. What this research revealed however that the impact of loneliness on psychological distress, including depression, was linked to self-perceptions of loneliness rather than objective measures of whether a person lived on their own. In the older sample questioned in one relevant study, some respondents lived on their own but they were not socially isolated from their families or friendship groups. Whether they lived alone or not made little or no difference to how likely they were to develop depression symptoms. What was more significant in this context was whether they felt they were isolated from social support groups. Those who "felt alone" were the ones more likely to get depressed (Taylor et al., 2018). Hence, even if people live alone, if steps can be taken to make them still feel connected, they do not invariably have to end up feeling "lonely".

Lockdown and Loneliness

The use of lockdowns during pandemics represents a class of interventions that can be deployed by governments and health authorities to control the spread of contagious viruses for which no effective pharmaceutical treatments are yet available. Applied effectively, they can control infection and more importantly, death rates from new diseases. Essentially, lockdowns are constructed around restrictions in physical and social contact between people.

Lockdowns built upon such stringent physical or social distancing measures, however, pose risks. They might offer some safeguards against infection from a new virus, but the restrictions they impose upon people in their everyday lives can cause health-related issues of their own. By prohibiting social connections, especially with loved ones, physical distancing rules might generate stresses that in turn cause mental health problems. Social isolation can lower people's moods and if this condition persists long enough, more serious chronic and debilitating health side-effects might follow on.

The closure of workplaces or requirements for employees to work exclusively from home is another intervention that is significant as far as tackling the spread of a highly infectious and mostly airborne virus, but also starves many people of regular social contact. The closure of universities meant that students could not enjoy normal campus experiences which were social as much as they were educational. School closures affected not only the educational progress of children but also represented a form of social deprivation and put pressure also on parents and carers expected to take some responsibility for the remote education of the children under their charge. In each case, the suspension of normal everyday activities for an ill-defined period of time put all those affected under considerable psychological strain which created harmful side-effects of its own.

Such restrictions can become particularly problematic psychologically for people when they are largely told to confine themselves to their homes and are not allowed to see members of their family or friends who live in different households. Such restrictions directly clash with a basic human need to socialise with others (Baumeister & Leary, 1995). Without regular social contact with others, especially those with whom we have close emotional ties, loneliness can set in and this can be a significant stressor that can trigger other health conditions (Hawkley & Cacioppo, 2010; Haslam et al., 2018). People might need this type of social support all the move during times of uncertainty and threat (Rimé, 2009; Jetten et al., 2012, Williams et al., 2018).

Experiencing this kind of social and sensory deprivation can prove to be very trying especially when the deprived have little space in which to move or must share their time between their usual workloads and new ones that are forced upon them by external circumstances beyond their control. Even when some social contact is permitted and possible, the removal of many of the amenities of everyday life that individuals take for granted can cause some people to re-think the meaning of their lives. This can be a positive experience for some and for others, not so much. Concern about the risks from a pandemic to self and others, worry about what the future holds and uncertainty about when normality will resume – if at all – can have profound effects on mood states.

Lockdown and Loneliness

Under the government's behavioural restrictions designed to combat the spread of the SARS-CoV-2 virus, social distancing was the cornerstone of each national lockdown. There was compulsory closure of most locations and spaces where people would normally interact physically and socially with each other. Many workplaces were closed as employees were encouraged to work from home. Places of hospitality and leisure venues, where people would socialise outside work, were also closed. This meant that there were few places open for people to go to. Essential shops that sold food, household products and medications remained open along with banks. Some coffee shops, cafes and restaurants and public houses remained open for takeaway and home delivery businesses. Hence, there were few opportunities for people to socialise. When rules were also introduced that prohibited people from socialising with people they did not live with, even in their own homes, most of the population was effectively placed under collective house arrest.

One of the major side-effect concerns about the physical distancing interventions deployed by governments to halt the spread of SARS-CoV-2 was loneliness. As people were required to isolate themselves physically and socially from others, they quickly missed the support they would normally from social companionship. Not only was this a painful consequence for many people, it was also known to be capable of giving rise to other more serious conditions, not least the deterioration of people's health – physical and mental (Holmes et al., 2020; Sanders, 2020). Not everyone experienced loneliness during the lockdown. Soundings taken during the first national lockdown in the United Kingdom between the end of March and mid-May 2020 found that although it was experienced by many to some degree, these symptoms were stronger among women than among men and among individuals aged 18–29 years and 3–59 years than among the 60s and over. Levels of loneliness among the 18–29s, however, decreased across this first lockdown and increased among the oldest adults (60+) (O'Connor et al., 2020).

Loneliness was already known to be linked to social deprivation, financial insecurity and poorer general health (Algren et al., 2020). The solution involves more than simply solving monetary problems. Ultimately, people need to interact with each other and establish close and supportive relationships. Take away social contact and deprive people of essential supportive experiences and there will eventually be adverse side effects. There are some social groups in society that are particularly at risk when their existing social contacts are switched off. These include people young and old who live alone and have limited family or social circles anyway. Those that live alone but normally have busy social lives with other single people can find social isolation especially difficult when they cannot enjoy their usual social lives because government restrictions prohibit people from different households intermingling (Algren et al., 2020).

Loneliness can create unpleasant feelings all by itself. Humans are social animals and when deprived of social contact, their lives can feel incomplete. It is not just that the immediate experience of being lonely is unpleasant, if it persists it can give rise to other problems. There is plenty of evidence from around the world that extreme social isolation can trigger ill-health conditions in the otherwise healthy and aggravate existing chronic health conditions (Steptoe, 2013; Holt-Lunstad, 2015; Santini, 2020). An association has been found between having poorly developed social networks and physical activity levels (Yu et al., 2011). Some research has shown that social isolation brings a significantly increased risk of dementia, heart disease and stroke and general mortality (Armitage & Nellums, 2020; Donovan, 2020). Isolation increases stress levels and these can in turn create greater anxiety, irritability, insomnia and depression (Brooks, 2020; Donovan, 2020; Holmes et al., 2020).

There are ways in which these adverse health effects can be mitigated. People need clarity about what is happening and indications of how long the extreme lockdown conditions will go on for. They need to discover meaningful activities to fill their days. They need to receive basic supplies of food, water and medications. Offline and online support can be used to provide these services and a sense of volunteering among the public will need to be created rather than a simple dependency on the government. One of the most profound responses to isolation is boredom and it is from this that a sense of hopelessness might emerge (Barari et al., 2020). Keeping people as connected as possible through whatever legitimate means remain available is critical in this context. By giving the "isolated" events to look forward to not only provides them with psychological reassurance that they are not alone but also lends some structure to their largely empty days.

Isolation and The Elderly

Isolation can be especially difficult for older people who were at greater risk of becoming seriously ill from COVID-19 (Luo et al., 2012). Having regular social contact can help to alleviate symptoms of loneliness among those already living alone. Persistent feelings of loneliness can disrupt the mental well-being of such people and aggravate physical health conditions that tend to become more chronic and prevalent with age (Cacioppo & Patrick 2009). Research in the United States among people aged 50+ showed that the restrictions that were imposed during the pandemic meant that many people became physically and socially isolated and this, in turn, increased feelings of loneliness, especially among those who felt most at risk from COVID-19. Some people used digital technologies to maintain some form of social contact, but this was not always enough to ensure that negative psychological side-effects were held at bay (Peng & Roth, 2021).

A major review of research from around the world showed international evidence for the mental health side-effects of social isolation on the elderly.

Isolation, among the elderly, could trigger anxiety symptoms, depression and sleep disorders (Sepúlveda-Loyola et al., 2020).

Isolation and Young People

Research emerged during the pandemic to show that the young experienced loneliness during the pandemic just as much as the elderly. Enforced separation from friends, disruption of social support networks and general uncertainty created a troubling psychological climate for young people (Walsh, 2021).

The impact of social isolation can also be profound even among younger people that are already isolated or suffering from ill-health conditions. Specific health conditions including cancer, heart disease, dementia and depression can be exacerbated by social isolation. The lack of close human contact can increase stress levels that compromise an individual's immune system and renders them more susceptible to worsening general health (Miller, 2020). Chapter 5 deals with the mental health effects of the pandemic among young people and Chapter 7 examines the impact of the pandemic on romantic and sexual relationships will shed further light on how youngsters were affected.

Isolation and The Unwell

Being deprived of social contact is bad enough if we are fit and well, but can be even more serious for those people who are already unwell. Research has shown that chronic social isolation can increase the risk of death from other ill-health conditions made worse by lack of human companionship and contact (Holt-Lunstad et al., 2010). For those individuals with serious health conditions, having regular social contact with others whom one knows one can rely on can significantly reduce mortality rates. This can be true in particular for patients returning home to recover from hospital treatments for serious health issues (Blazer, 1982; Forster & Stoller, 1992; Wang et al., 2005; Murphy et al., 2008).

The damaging effects of social isolation can be profound even among people who already live alone. Those individuals from single-person households might still enjoy the company of others from elsewhere. Under the pandemic lockdown restrictions, however, meetings between people from different households were prohibited even though those visitors might be next-of-kin. These links can be particularly important to older people who were the most affected by lockdown restrictions simply because they were classed as most at risk from COVID-19.

Public Responses to Lockdown

Ipsos-MORI conducted research for the Academy of Sciences and the mental health charity, MQ to investigate early in the pandemic in the UK people's perceptions of the impact it was having on their mental well-being. It also enquired into what people had been doing to tackle this issue. Over 1,000 people were questioned, aged 16–75 years, between 26th and 30th March, just a few days after full lockdown had been implemented (Worsley & Williams, 2020, 16th April).

One in five people questioned (21%) were already concerned about being placed in social isolation and a similar proportion (18%) had concerns about not being able to go out freely as often and wherever they liked. A few people specifically said they were concerned about social distancing (13%) and there were low-level signs at this point of concerns about the lack of social contact (5%) and loneliness (4%). One in five (20%) expressed concerns about the impact of the lockdown on mental illnesses. Whether this was a generic concern for society or more specifically for themselves was not totally made clear here, but a few were concerned about anxiety (11%) and depression (7%). There were gender differences here and in particular women (28%) were far more likely than men (13%) to express concern about mental illnesses.

What did people do to counter these concerns? One in four (24%) turned to various forms of entertainment that included reading do-it-yourself and listening to music. One in five (22%) did their best to keep in touch with family and friends through electronic means such as video calls and social media sites. Other activities that seemed to help a few included household chores, working from home and getting outside when they could.

King's College London and Ipsos-MORI interviewed 2,250 people across the United Kingdom aged 18–75 between 1st and 3rd April 2020. This survey found that on average people that were questioned said they could probably manage to cope with lockdown for up to six weeks, but after that, they felt that things could then get more difficult. One in seven (15%) reported already experiencing difficulties coping. Young people aged 16–24 (42%) were the most likely to report early difficulties coping with lockdown (King's College London, 2020, 9th April).

Despite the fact that many people missed normality after only a couple of weeks without it, a substantial minority (41%) recognised that coronavirus interventions could last for many months. More than half (51%) even thought that it might take over a year before life could return to normal. There was no doubt about the seriousness of the virus in people's minds with over four in ten (43%) predicting at least 20,000 COVID-19-related deaths and one in ten (11%) believing deaths could exceed 100,000. Given these early depressing perceptions of the crisis, it was little surprise that a sizeable proportion of the people interviewed here (49%) reported feeling more anxious or depressed than normal. Nearly four in ten (38%) said they had slept less well.

Happiness and Mental Health: Lockdown Effects

Despite the lockdown triggering debates about its negative impact on the mental health of the nation, evidence emerged that for at least some people, a period of temporary social isolation had actually improved their subjective well-being. This observation was supported by research evidence reported by pollster, YouGov, working in partnership with the University of Cambridge. Researchers working at the Bennett Institute for Public Policy analysed data from YouGov surveys and Google searches to track the well-being of people in Britain.

The picture was quite a bit different at the beginning of lockdown, however, using YouGov happiness tracking data, findings showed that the proportion of British people saying they were "happy" reached just over half (51%) about a month before lockdown and fell dramatically (to 25%) as lockdown began, By the end of May 2020, however, happiness levels had almost returned to their pre-lockdown position (47%) (Rogers de Waal, 2020, 1st August).

The evidence was interpreted as showing that the pandemic did have a negative impact on mental well-being, but that this had occurred even before full lockdowns were put in place by governments. Once a wide range of non-pharmaceutical interventions had been put in place, people eventually snapped out of their malaise as these lockdowns wore on (Foa et al., 2020).

Concerns were raised about the effects of being locked down on people's mental health. Various experts raised the possibility, backed up by scientific evidence that draconian measures designed to restrict social contact between people could create a wave of loneliness especially among those already on their own which could lead, in turn, to anxiety and depression (Brooks et al., 2020; Courtet et al., 2020). The research was released early in lockdowns to show that these symptoms were being registered among vulnerable people in Britain. The pandemic had triggered a decline in mental health not just among some people in the United Kingdom but also as far afield as China and New Zealand (Banks & Xu, 2020; Cao et al., 2020; Sibley et al., 2020; Zhang et al., 2020).

Yet, these findings were not replicated everywhere. Even within the United Kingdom, research emerged to show that anxiety and depression had not grown worse across the lockdown (Fancourt et al., 2021). Similarly, in the United States, further evidence emerged being lockdown did not make everyone feel lonely (Luchetti et al., 2020). There was evidence that the restrictions of lockdown did leave some people feeling very bored and therefore also saddened to some extent by not being able to pursue specific activities they enjoyed (Brodeur et al., 2020). In locations such as Paris, for example, where many people lived in small apartments with little outdoor space, being required to remain indoors did give rise to negative mood states for many (Recchi et al., 2020).

One important question that was frequently not answered by the initial research was whether negative mood states were triggered specifically by the lockdown or whether they represented a more general reaction to the pandemic. It is possible that the existence of the pandemic with the threats it posed to personal health and well-being was a distinctive causal factor affecting public mood (Cao et al., 2020; Gao et al., 2020; Zhang et al., 2020). On top of this, lockdown interventions could have contributed further to how people felt. Lockdowns tended to comprise a range of non-pharmaceutical interventions that could impact upon people's lives in different ways. Specific interventions could be profound in their effects for some people, but not so much for others. A person living alone in a one-bedroom apartment with no outdoor space might have a radically different experience of a lockdown that required everyone to stay home from, say, someone living with several family members in a detached house with a large garden.

Hence, in understanding the mental health impact of the pandemic and lockdown measures, research methodologies are needed that separate out pandemic-specific effects and lockdown-specific effects and also differentiate between different people according to their living and life circumstances and conditions. The studies cited above did not make these distinctions. Furthermore, when measuring mood and other health-related effects, physical and mental symptoms need to be distinctively defined and measured (Layard et al., 2020). Only when this type of finer-grained data are available can properly be informed lockdown-release decisions be implemented that consider in a more carefully targeted fashion, the specific links between different interventions and specific health outcomes.

In a large web survey of households that had taken part in the United Kingdom Household Longitudinal Study, members aged 16 and over provided evidence on their mental state one month after lockdown had started (23rd–30th April 2020). There was an increased prevalence of clinically measured levels of mental distress in April 2020 (27%) compared to a year earlier (19%). Not only had measures of general mental health indicated a continuation of the upward trend observed over the previous six years, but the year-on-year increase observed during the coronavirus pandemic lockdown also exhibited an accelerated rate of increase. Put simply, the lockdown had triggered greater levels of mental stress and anxiety than normal and pushed up their overall prevalence to a greater extent than would otherwise have been anticipated. Bear in mind also, that this initial sounding took place just one into lockdown (Pierce et al., 2020).

This greater than expected rise in mental distress across the British population was not evenly distributed, but varied in prevalence between sub-groups. This finding was not new and reflected in broad terms what was expected from previous findings, which had shown mental distress prevalence to vary by age, gender, socio-economic status, general mental and physical health status and household type. The 2020 lockdown findings indicated that those experiencing the worst mental health outcomes tended to be young, female and lived with children, especially preschool-age children. Before lockdown, the highest rates of mental distress were found amongst the unemployed and full-time students. During the lockdown, however, it was the employed that experienced significant shifts in the prevalence of stress and anxiety as their jobs were lost or put under serious threat, or as a result of having to adapt to home-working or working out of home in situations that put them under threat of infection from COVID-19.

The findings did not confirm other hypothesised changes in mental distress levels linked to other pre-existing characteristics. Hence, they found no significant changes in mental state for ethnic minorities, those living in inner-city areas, being unemployed or having a health condition that made a person at higher risk of coronavirus infection. Once again, though, the researchers pointed out that these soundings were taken after only one month of lockdown. In the longer term, the mental health costs of these government interventions into people's working and private lives might be expected to spread farther and wider. A longer lockdown or repeated lockdown releases and closures could have significant economic costs for many people that would in turn pose serious risks to their mental health.

The research was conducted in April 2020, during the first six weeks of lockdown, to examine how people initially responded to the lockdown measures implemented by the UK government. A sample of adults aged 18 and over was recruited via social media between 3rd April and 30th April 2020 for a survey examining the consequences of the coronavirus lockdown on people's mental health (Jia et al., 2020). This was not a representative sample, which limits the generalisability of its findings to people in general, and much of the sample of volunteers was female with an average age of 4 years. Half of the respondents described themselves as key workers and one in five claimed to have clinical risk factors putting them at increased risk from COVID-19.

At the time of the study, there was still much to be learned about this new coronavirus, but already early signs had emerged that taking extreme measures to tackle its spread could have profound spin-off physical and mental health side-effects (Candan et al., 2020). Further evidence concerning earlier pandemics had previously indicated that severe non-pharmaceutical interventions could have a range of serious health consequences (Chan et al., 2006; Jeong et al., 2016; Liu et al., 2020; Tian et al., 2020).

Initial evidence for the United Kingdom had already shown that the health side-effects observed in Asia, where previous pandemics had hit, could be replicated (Williams et al., 2020). It was also discovered early on that certain groups were more at risk than others of serious illness once infected by this new virus and this also opened up the possibility that these groups might also be at greater risk of psychological side-effects. Hence, older people, men and members of black and minority ethnic communities were found to be at greater risk of hospitalisation and death from COVID-19 (Office of National Statistics, 2020, 20th April; Zhou et al., 2020).

The Health Foundation found that by early May 2020, three-quarters of people (77%) across Great Britain were concerned about the health impact on the nation of social distancing measures (The Health Foundation, 2020, June). This opinion was even more widely held among the over-65s (83%). Nearly half of people (47%) said they were finding it difficult to communicate with family and friends. Over half (54%) claimed they were having problems getting basic food items and nearly half (46%) felt that the crisis was affecting their mental health. Four in ten (41%) had lost income because of the pandemic and quite a few had had to dip into their savings (17%) or take-out loans (12%) to survive. People were therefore clearly under a lot of economic and psychological pressure.

Another concern about psychological reactions and their further impact on an individual's health status was that some individuals might be more prone to perceive the personal risk of COVID-19 infection and greater associated anxiety about becoming seriously ill in consequence. Such psychological states were known to dampen down immune responses if they were pronounced and persistent. Hence, as well as the effects of worry on the person's own mental well-being, there could be a further impact on their physical health (Salkovskis et al., 2002; Bults et al., 2011; Gao et al., 2020). Physical or social distancing produced extreme social isolation for some people generating feelings of loneliness that caused further stress and anxiety. For individuals who were already isolated, this could create further difficulties if their usual limited support networks were disrupted. For those used to regular social companionship, but who nevertheless lived alone, being cut off from regular social contact could be extremely distressing. Once again, there is an important psychological dimension linked to self-perception in this context that can have profound health consequences.

People who perceive themselves as lacking support and as being lonely can experience mental health problems that generally raise their risk of becoming seriously ill when exposed to infections (Leigh-Hunt et al., 2017; Wang et al., 2018). People with positive mood states tend to be healthier and have more robust immune responses when exposed to infections (Folkman, 1997; Larsen et al., 2017; Pressman et al., 2019). Hence, keeping in a good mood and an upbeat frame of mind not only reduces anxiety and related psychological disorders, but also renders the individual as physically and mentally more robust, helping them to avoid infections and aiding recovery if they are unfortunate enough to become infected (Schotanus-Dijkstra et al., 2017, 2019).

The research by Jia and his colleagues found that their sample reported anxiety and depression symptoms to a greater extent than previous studies had revealed for British people, based on more representative samples

(Löwe et al., 2008; Kocalevent et al., 2013; Warttig et al., 2013). These findings appeared for both women and men in the sample, but was characteristic more of people aged under 65. Older people in this sample exhibited anxiety scores more consistent with those found for larger and more representative samples. It is worth bearing in mind here that a significant proportion of respondents in this early lockdown survey were front-line healthcare workers.

The inflated anxiety and depression scores could therefore have been indicative of the stress they were under as they were coping with the peak of the first wave of the pandemic. In fact, nearly two-thirds of the sample (64%) reported symptoms of depression and over half (57%) reported anxiety. Severe depressive symptoms were reported by over three in ten respondents (31%) and severe anxiety symptoms by one in four (26%). Further analysis of how these psychological symptoms varied between different sub-groups in the sample showed, however, that being a frontline healthcare worker was not a significant predictor of anxiety and depression. More important was being female and also being within a COVID-19 "at-risk" group. People who thought they were at great risk of catching the disease and that if they did so they would die from it, understandably became anxious about it.

Being more stressed by COVID-19 and the lockdown was greater among younger people, women, people that lived alone, being from a BAME background and being from an identified at-risk group. There was some evidence that being a key worker was a predictor factor for stress, but was actually associated with *lower* stress scores.

It is important to note that the data used here to measure depression, anxiety and stress derived from self-assessments made by respondents on psychological scales distributed via questionnaire. These self-reports were not separately clinically validated by relevant medical experts. Nonetheless, the psychological tests had been developed to enable people to make their own self-assessments and these tests had been previously validated for their clinical insights (Löwe et al., 2008; Kocalevent et al., 2013; Warttig, et al., 2013).

Search for Coping Mechanisms

Being placed in involuntary social isolation and, if infected, home arrest, meant that many people found themselves with time on their hands with little to do. For those able to work from home, this was not such a problem. For those parents and carers landed with home schooling, many found themselves with more on their hands than they bargained for. Yet, for many people, the absence of places to go and restrictions on who they could meet up with meant that they were starved of structure to their lives and social contact. This state of affairs left some feeling lonely and, as we will see in the next chapter, some also experienced more serious mental health side effects. Eventually, many sought out new ways of filling their time and in this context, the entertainment media provided popular distractions from the threat of this new disease and the tedium of lockdown.

One of the key concerns linked to loneliness is that it can leave sufferers vulnerable to other psychological problems. Frequently, these other problems are driven by unhappiness that stems from feeling alone. It is important to recognise that *being* alone is not the same as *feeling* alone. The former is a physical state and the latter is a psychological state (Julie-Deniere, 2020). Some people might choose to be on their own for temporary periods or even to live that way because psychologically and socially it suits them. Being on their own will not usually make these people feel lonely. As we have seen, being happy is important in promoting good mental and physical health. Being lonely – that is feeling alone for reasons not of the individual's own making – can produce loss of happiness or sadness. If this mood still persists, it can bring the individual down and result in more chronic ill-health including traumatic stress feelings and depression. This issue is examined in more detail in the next chapter. In the meantime, it is possible to empower individuals to combat isolation and loneliness. If techniques with this end in mind can be taught and successfully deployed, then chronic and long-term ill-health could be avoided or its effects reduced.

In the modern technological world, young people spend increasing amounts of time online and this forms an important part of their social lives. This also means that they can be on their own as a physical state, but still remain in contact with others remotely via various communications technologies. During the pandemic, people around the world had to contend with behavioural restrictions imposed upon them by their governments. In terms of physical states, these restrictions meant that many people were deprived of social contact, especially if they lived on their own. Even those who lived with someone were often restricted to social contact only with that one individual. Hence, the conditions were created in which loneliness – or feeling alone – could develop as a state of being, unless individuals were accustomed to *being alone* while not *being lonely* because they had integrated remote contact methods into their social lives.

Loneliness is not an immovable state. There are coping techniques that anyone can adopt to reduce their feelings of loneliness. In part, this entails removing negative thoughts about being alone. It also entails taking positive action such as arranging to go out to places where there are other people and where there are opportunities to engage with them (Leahy, 2017).

During the pandemic, the most extreme regimes of behavioural restrictions, often referred to as "lockdowns", meant that individuals were not allowed to go out to meet others from different households. Nevertheless, social contacts could still be maintained through video links. Another therapeutic technique is for an individual to recognise that when they feel lonely, as they might during a pandemic lockdown, their negative feelings are often triggered by a critical internal "voice" that tells them that being alone is bad and sad. They need to separate this critical voice from their true self, and one way of doing this is to write down what this inner critic is saying and then finding counter-arguments with a more positive tone that seeks solutions to their current loos of happiness (Firestone, 2020).

Research evidence emerged from Canada and the United States that the media could serve as sources of psychological coping mechanisms. People across North America reported new media habits and experiences once the COVID-19 outbreak had kicked in (Pahayahay & Khalili-Mahani, 2020). People who admitted that their mental health was not good exhibited a propensity to watch streamed services on TV to deal with social isolation. Women and non-binary respondents were much more likely than men as a coping method for dealing with social isolation. Respondents aged under 35 were most likely to name computer games while the over 55s were more likely to watch network TV or read newspapers to cope with changed circumstances. Follow-up qualitative research with respondents in which they had more scope to articulate their media habits in detail showed the mainstream media and social media could provide support through their factual information about COVID-19, especially if it was positive and also countered or helped them to avoid or discount fake news and mis-information, which tended to be more negative.

In closing, there was ample evidence that widespread public fear spread through many populations at the start of the pandemic as national governments imposed restrictions that were unprecedented in most people's lifetimes. There was a climate of uncertainty about how long the pandemic would last and how much danger it posed to individuals should they become ill. As science learned rapid lessons about the new virus, some of these fears were allayed. Yet, the dramatic suspension of normal life for virtually everyone reminded people of how quickly everyday conditions that everyone took for granted could be taken away almost overnight. Some people found ways of adapting to these changed circumstances. For some, it caused them to reflect on the ways they lived their lives and triggered thoughts about alternative lifestyles. For some, however, their initial and natural fear responses to the threatening circumstances of which they were constantly reminded everyday by the media and conversations with others, transformed into more chronic mental health states. For these individuals, for whom psychological coping mechanisms had eluded them, the pandemic caused considerable personal collateral damage. This book will turn in the chapters ahead to the different forms in which this collateral damage was manifest.

References

Algren, M. H., Ekholm, O., Nielsen, L., Ersbøll, A. K., Bak, C. K., & Andersen, P. T. (2020). Social isolation, loneliness, socioeconomic status, and health-risk behaviour in deprived neighbourhoods in Denmark: A cross-sectional study. *SSM Population Health*, 10: 100546. doi:10.1016/j.ssmph.2020.100546

Armitage, R., & Nellums, L. B. (2020). COVID-19 and the consequences of isolating the elderly. *The Lancet*, 5(5): E256. doi: https://www.doi.org/10.1016/S24 68-2667(20)30061-x

Banks, J. & Xu, X. (2020). The mental health effects of the first two months of lockdown and social distancing during the COVID-19 pandemic in the UK.' *IFS Working Paper*, 20/16. London, UK: Institute for Fiscal Studies. Retrieved from: https://ifs.org.uk/uploads/WP202016-Covid-and-mental-health.pdf

Barari, S., Caria, S., Davola, A., Falco, P., Fetzer, T., et al. (2020). Evaluating COVID-18 public health messaging in Italy: Self-reported compliance and growing mental health concerns. *MedRxiv*. doi: 10.1101/2020.03.27.20042820

Beaver, K. (2020, 30th July). Face masks becoming normal but flashpoint while 'COVID-secure' behaviours sticking. Ipsos-MORI. Available at: https://www.ipsos. com/ipsos-mori/en-uk/face-masks-becoming-normal-flashpoint-while-covid-secure-behaviours-sticking

Baumeister, R. F. & Leary, M. R. (1995). The need to belong: Desire for interpersonal attachments as a fundamental human motivation. *Psychological Bulletin*, 117: 497–529.

Blazer, D. G. (1982). Social support and mortality in an elderly community population. *American Journal of Epidemiology*, 115: 684–694.

Brodeur, A., Clark, A. E., Fleche, S. & Powdthavee, N. (2020). COVID-19, lockdowns and well-being: Evidence from Google Trends. *IZA Discussion Paper #13204*. Bonn, Germany: Institute of Labour Economics. Retrieved from: https://www.iza. org/publications/dp/13204/covid-19-lockdowns-and-well-being-evidence-from-google-trends

Brooks, S. K., Webster, R. J., Smith, L. E., Woodland, L., Wessely, S., & Greenberg, N. (2020). The psychological impact of quarantine and how to reduce it: Rapid review of the evidence. *The Lancet*, 395: 912–920.

Brooks, S. K., Webster, R. K., Smith, L. E., Woodland, L., Wessely, S., Greenberg, N. & Rubin, J. G. (2020). The psychological impact of quarantine and how to reduce it: Rapid review of the evidence. *The Lancet*, 395(1022): 912–920.

Bults, M., Beaujean, D. J., de Zwart, O., Kok, G., van Empelen, P., van Steenbergen, J. E., Richardus, J. H., & Voeten, H. A. (2011). Perceived risk, anxiety, and behavioural responses of the general public during the early phase of the Influenza A (H1N1) pandemic in the Netherlands: Results of three consecutive online surveys. *BMC Public Health*, 11: 2. doi: 10.1186/1471-2458-11-2

Bulkeley, K. (2020, 12th April). Common themes in dreams about the pandemic. Psychology Today. Retrieved from: https://www.psychologytoday.com/gb/blog/dreaming-in-the-digital-age/202004/common-themes-in-dreams-about-the-pandemic

Cacioppo, J. T., Cacioppo, S., Capitanio, J. P., & Cole, S. W. (2015). The neuroendocrinology of social isolation. *Annual Review of Psychology*, 66: 733–767. doi: 10.1146/annurev-psych-010814-015240

Cacioppo, J. T., & Hawkley, L. C. (2003). Social isolation and health, with an emphasis on underlying mechanisms. *Perspectives in Biology and Medicine*, 46: S39–S52. doi: 10.1353/pbm.2003.0049

Cacioppo, J. T. & Patrick, W. (2009). *Loneliness: Human Nature and the Need for Social Connection*. London, UK: W. W. Norton & Co.

Candan, S. A., Elibol, N., & Abdullahi, A. (2020). Consideration of prevention and management of long-term consequences of post-acute respiratory distress syndrome in patients with COVID-19. *Physiotherapy Theory and Practice*, 36(6): 663–668. doi: 10.1080/09593985.2020.1766181

Cao, W., Fang, Z., Hou, G., Han, M., Xu, X., Dong, J., & Zheng, J. (2020). The Psychological Impact of the COVID-19 Epidemic on College Students in China. *Psychiatry Research*, 287(112934): 1–5.

Chan, S. M., Chiu, F. K., Lam, C. W., Leung, P. Y., & Conwell, Y. (2006). Elderly suicide and the 2003 SARS epidemic in Hong Kong. *International Journal of Geriatric Psychiatry*, 21(2): 113–118. doi: 10.1002/gps.1432

Courtet, P., Olie, E., Debien, C., & Vaiva, G. (2020). Keep socially (but not physically) connected and carry on: Preventing suicide in the age of COVID-19. *Journal of Clinical Psychiatry*, 81(3): e1–e3.

Crisell, H. (2020, 8th June). Covid dreams: How strange are yours? *The Times: Times 2*, 2: 2–3.

Daly, M., & Robinson, E. (2021). Psychological distress and adaptation to the COVID-19 crisis in the United States. *Journal of Psychiatric Research*, 136: 603–609. doi: 10.1016/j.jpsychires.2020.10.035

Donovan, N. J. (2020). Timely insights into the treatment of social disconnection in lonely, homebound older adults. *The American Journal of Geriatric Psychiatry*, 28(7): 709–711.

Fancourt, D., Steptoe, A., & Bu, F. (2021). Trajectories of anxiety and depressive symptoms during enforced isolation due to COVID-19 in England: a longitudinal observational study. *Lancet Psychiatry*, 8(2): 141–149. doi: 10.1016/S2215-0366(20)30482-X

Firestone, L. (2020, 20th April). Coping with loneliness during a pandemic. *Psychology Today*. Retrieved from: https://www.psychologytoday.com/gb/blog/compassion-matters/202004/coping-loneliness-during-pandemic

Foa, R. S., Gilbert, S., & Fabian, M. O. (2020). *Covid-19 and Subjective Well-being: Separating Effects of Lockdowns from the Pandemic*. Cambridge, MA: Bennett Institute for Public Policy. Retrieved fromt: https://www.bennettinstitute.cam.ac.uk/publications/covid-19-and-subjective-well-being/ 2nd September 2020.

Folkman, S. (1997). Positive psychological states and coping with severe stress. *Social Science and Medicine*, 45(8): 1207–1221. doi: 10.1016/s0277-9536(97)00040-3

Forster, L. E., & Stoller, E. P. (1992). The impact of social support on mortality: A seven-year follow-up of older men and women. *Journal of Applied Gerontology*, 11: 173–186.

Gao, J., Zheng, P., Jia, Y., Chen, H., Mao, Y., Chen, S., Wang, Y., Fu, H., & Dai, J. (2020). Mental health problems and social media exposure during COVID-19 Outbreak.' *PLoS ONE*, 15(4): 1–10.

Haslam, C., Jetten, J., Cruwys, T., Dingle, G., & Haslam, S. A. (2018). *The New Psychology of Health: Unlocking the Social Cure*. London, UK: Routledge.

Hawkley, L. C. & Cacioppo, J. T. (2010). Loneliness matters: a theoretical and empirical review of consequences and mechanisms. *Annals of Behavioural Medicine*, 40: 218–227.

Holt-Lunstad, J. (2015). Loneliness and social isolation as risk factors for mortality: A meta-analytic review. *Perspectives in Psychological Science*, 10(2): 227–237.

Holt-Lunstad, J., & Smith, T. B. (2016). Loneliness and social isolation as risk factors for CVD: Implications for evidence-based patient care and scientific enquiry. *Heart*, 102: 987–989.

Holt-Lunstad, J., Smith, T. B., & Layton, J. B. (2010). Social relationships and mortality risk: A meta-analytic review. *PLoS Medicine*, 7(7): e1000316.

Holt-Lunstad, J., Smith, T. B., Baker, M., Harris, T., & Stephenson, D. (2015). Loneliness and social isolation as risk factors for mortality: A meta-analysis review. *Perspectives on Psychological Science: A Journal of the Association for Psychological Science*, 10(2): 227–237.

Holmes, E. A., O'Connor, R. C., Perry, V. H., Tracey, I., Wesseley, S., Arsenault, L., et al. (2020). Multidisciplinary research priorities for the COVID-19 pandemic: A call for action for mental health science. *Lancet Psychiatry*, 7(6): 547–560.

Jeong, H., Yim, H. W., Song, Y. J., Ki, M., Min, J. A., Cho, J., & Chae, J. H. (2016). Mental health status of people isolated due to Middle East Respiratory Syndrome. *Epidemiology and Health*, 5(38): e2016048. doi: 10.4178/epih.e2016048

Jetten, J., Haslam, C., & Haslam, S. A. (Eds.) (2012). The Social Cure: Identity, Health and Well-being. Psychology Press.

Jia, R., Ayling, K., Chalder, T., Massy, A., Broadbent, E., Coupland, C., & Vedhara, K. (2020). Mental health in the UK during the COVID-19 pandemic: Cross-sectional analyses from a community cohort study. *BMJ Open*, 10(9). Available at: https://bmjopen.bmj.com/content/bmjopen/10/9/e040620.full.pdf

Julie-Deniere, E. (2020, 16th April). Being alone vs being lonely. *Psychology Today*. Retrieved from: https://www.psychologytoday.com/gb/blog/talking-emotion/202004/being-alone-vs-being-lonely

King's College London (2020, 9th April). Life under lockdown: coronavirus in the UK. Available at: https://www.kcl.ac.uk/news/life-under-lockdown-coronavirus-in-the-uk

Kocalevent, R. D., Hinz, A., & Brähler, E. (2013). Standardization of a screening instrument (PHQ-15) for somatization syndromes in the general population. *BMC Psychiatry*, 20(13): 91. doi: 10.1186/1471-244X-13-91

Lara, E., Martin-Marla, N., de la Torre-Luque, A., Koyanago, A., Vancampfort, D., Izquierdo, A., & Meret, M. (2019). Does loneliness contribute to mild cognitive impairment and dementia? A systematic review and meta-analysis of longitudinal studies. *Ageing Research Reviews*, 52: 7–16.

Larsen, J. T., Hershfield, H., Stastny, B. J., & Hester, N. (2017). On the relationship between positive and negative affect: Their correlation and their co-occurrence. *Emotion*, 17: 323–336. 10.1037/ emo0000231

Layard, R., A. Clark, J.-E. De Neve, C. Krekel, D. Fancourt, N. Hey, & G. O'Donnell, "When to release the lockdown: A wellbeing framework for analysing costs and benefits," *CEP Occasional Paper*, 49, 2020. Retrieved: https://blogs.lse.ac.uk/covid19/2020/05/13/when-to-release-the-lockdown-a-wellbeing-framework-for-analysing-costs-and-benefits/

Leahy, R. L. (2017, 9th February). Living with loneliness. *Psychology Today*. Retrieved from: https://www.psychologytoday.com/gb/blog/anxiety-files/201702/living-loneliness

Leigh-Hunt, N., Bagguley, D., Bash, K., Turner, V., Turnbull, S., Valtorta, N., & Caan, W. (2017). An overview of systematic reviews on the public health consequences of social isolation and loneliness. *Public Health*, 152: 157–171. doi: 10.1016/j.puhe.2017.07.035

Liu, S., Yang, L., Zhang, C., Xiang, Y. T., Liu, Z., Hu, S., & Zhang, B. (2020). Online mental health services in China during the COVID-19 outbreak. *Lancet Psychiatry*, 7(4): e17–e18. doi: 10.1016/S2215-0366(20)30077-8

Löwe, B., Decker, O., Müller, S., Brähler, E., Schellberg, D., Herzog, W., & Herzberg, P. Y. (2008). Validation and standardization of the Generalized Anxiety Disorder Screener (GAD-7) in the general population. *Medical Care*, 46(3): 266–274. doi: 10.1097/MLR.0b013e318160d093

Luchetti, M., Lee, J. H., Aschwanden, D., Sesker, A., Strickhouser, J., Terracciano, A. & Sutin, A. (2020). The trajectory of loneliness in response to COVID-19. *American Psychologist*, 75(7): 897–908. doi: 10.1037/amp0000690

Luo, Y., Hawkley, L. C., Waite, L. J., & Cacioppo, J. T. (2012). Loneliness, health, and mortality in old age: a national longitudinal study. *Soc. Sci. Med*, 74: 907–914.

McAndrew, F. T. (2016, 12th November). The perils of social isolation. *Psychology Today*. https://www.psychologytoday.com/us/blog/out-the-ooze/201611/the-perils-of-social-isolation

Mental Health Foundation (2020a, 9th July). Coronavirus: The divergence of mental health experiences during the pandemic. Retrieved from: https://www.mentalhealth.org.uk/coronavirus/divergence-mental-health-experiences-during-pandemic

Mental Health Foundation (2020b, 8th October). Resilience across the UK during the coronavirus pandemic. Available at: https://www.mentalhealth.org.uk/coronavirus/resilience-across-uk-coronavirus-pandemic

Miller, G. (2020, 16th March). Social distancing prevents infections, but it can have unintended consequences. *Science*. Available at: www.science.org/news/2020/03/we-are-social-species-how-will-social-distancing-affect-us

Murphy, B. M., Elliott, P. C., Le Grande, M. R., Higgins, R. O., Ernest, C. S. et al. (2008). Living alone predicts 30-day hospital readmission after coronary artery bypass graft surgery. *European Journal of Cardiovascular Preventive Rehabilitation*, 15: 210–215.

O'Connor, R. C., Wetherall, K., Cleare, S., McClelland, H., Melson, A. J., Niedzwiedz, C. L., O'Carroll, R. E., O'Connor, D. B., Platt, S., Scowcroft, E., Watson, B., Zortea, T., Ferguson, E., & Robb, K. A. (2020). Mental health and well-being during the COVID-19 pandemic: longitudinal analyses of adults in the UK COVID-19 Mental Health & Wellbeing study. *British Journal of Psychiatry*, 21: 1–8. doi: 10.1192/bjp.2020.212

Office for National Statistics. (2020, 20th April). Coronavirus (COVID-19) related deaths by occupation, England and Wales: deaths registered up to and including 20 April 2020. Retrieved from: https://www.ons.gov.uk/releases/covid19relateddeathsbyoccupationenglandandwalesdeathsregistereduptoandincluding20thapril2020

Pahayahay, A. & Khalili-Mahani, N. (2020). What media helps, what media hurts: A mixed methods survey study of coping with COVID-19 using the media repertoire framework and the appraisal theory of stress. *Journal of Medicine and Internet Research*, 22(8): e21086. Doi:10.2196/20186

Peng, S. & Roth, A. R. (2021). Social isolation and loneliness before and during the COVID-19 pandemic: A longitudinal study of U.S. adults older than 50, *The Journals of Gerontology: Series B*, gbab068, 10.1093/geronb/gbab068

Pierce, M., Hope, H., Ford, T., Hatch, S., Hotopf, M., & John, A. (2020). Mental health before and during the COVID-19 pandemic: a longitudinal probability sample survey of the UK population. *The Lancet Psychiatry*, 7(10): 883–892.

Pressman, S. D., Jenkins, B. N., & Moskowitz, J. T. (2019). Positive affect and health: What do we know and where next should we go? *Annual Review of Psychology*, 70: 627–650. doi: 10.1146/annurev-psych-010418-102955

Renner, R. (2020, 15th April). The pandemic is giving people vivid, unusual dreams. Here's why. *National Geographic*. Retrieved from: https://www.nationalgeographic.co.uk/science-and-technology/2020/04/pandemic-giving-people-vivid-unusual-dreams-heres-why

Recchi, E., Ferragina, E., Helmeid, E., Pauly, S., Sa., M., Sauger, N., & Schradie, J. (2020). The `eye of the hurricane' paradox: An unexpected and unequal rise of well-being during the COVID-19 lockdown in France. *Research in Social Stratification and Mobility*, 68: 100508. doi: 10.1016/j.rssm.2020.100508

Rimé, B. (2009). Emotion elicits the social sharing of emotion: Theory and empirical review. *Emotion Reviews*, 1: 60–85.

Rogers de Waal, J. (2020, 1st August). Lockdown led to happiness rebound. YouGov. Available at: https://yougov.co.uk/topics/health/articles-reports/2020/08/01/lockdown-led-happiness-rebound-according-yougov-ca 2nd September 2020.

Rushby-Jones, K. (2020, 21st July). Loneliness is lethal. *The Psychologist*. Retrieved from: https://thepsychologist.bps.org.uk/loneliness-lethal

Salkovskis, P. M., Rimes, K. A., Warwick, H. M., & Clark, D. M. (2002). The Health Anxiety Inventory: Development and validation of scales for the measurement of health anxiety and hypochondriasis. *Psychological Medicine*, 32(5): 843–853. doi: 10.1017/s0033291702005822

Sanders, R. (2020, 22nd April). COVID-19, social isolation and loneliness. Iriss. Available at: https://www.iriss.org.uk/resources/esss-outlines/covid-19-social-isolation-amd-loneliness

Santini, Z. (2020). Social disconnectedness, perceived isolation and symptoms of depression and anxiety among older Americans: a longitudinal mediation analysis. *Lancet Public Health*, 5(1): e62–e70.

Schotanus-Dijkstra, M., Ten Have, M., Lamers, S. M. A., de Graaf, R., & Bohlmeijer, E. T. (2017). The longitudinal relationship between flourishing mental health and incident mood, anxiety and substance use disorders. *European Journal of Public Health*, 27(3): 563–568. doi: 10.1093/eurpub/ckw202

Schotanus-Dijkstra, M., Keyes, C. L. M., de Graaf, R., & Ten Have, M. (2019). Recovery from mood and anxiety disorders: The influence of positive mental health. *Journal of Affective Disorders*, 1(252): 107–113. doi: 10.1016/j.jad.2019.04.051

Sepúlveda-Loyola, W., Rodríguez-Sánchez, I., Pérez-Rodríguez, P., Ganz, F., Torralba, R., Oliveira, D. V., & Rodríguez-Mañas, L. (2020). Impact of social isolation due to COVID-19 on health in older people: mental and physical effects and recommendations. *The Journal of Nutrition, Health & Aging*, 1–10. 10.1007/s12603-020-1469-2

Sibley, C. G., Greaves, L. M., Satherley, N., Wilson, M. S., Overall, N. C. , Lee, C. et al. (2020). Effects of the COVID-19 pandemic and nationwide lockdown on trust, attitudes towards government, and well-being. *American Psychologist*, 75(5): 618–630. doi: 10.1037/amp0000662

Steptoe, A. (2013). Social isolation, loneliness, and all-cause mortality in older men and women. *Proceedings of the National Academy of Science of the USA*, 110(15): 5797–5801.

Taylor, H. O., Taylor, R. J., Nguyen, A. W., & Chatters, L. (2018). Social isolation, depression and psychological distress among older adults. *Journal of Aging and Health*, 30(2): 229–246.

The Health Foundation (2020, June). Public perceptions of health and social care in light of COVID-19 (May 2020) Available at: https://www.health.org.uk/publications/reports/public-perceptions-of-health-and-social-care-in-light-of-covid-19-may-2020

Thomson, A. (2020, 21st October). Second wave is bringing a mental health crisis. *The Times*, p. 25.

Tian, H., Liu, Y., Li, Y., Wu, C. H., Chen, B., Kraemer, M. U. G., Li, B., Cai, J., Xu, B., Yang, Q., Wang, B., Yang, P., Cui, Y., Song, Y., Zheng, P., Wang, Q., Bjornstad, O. N., Yang, R., Grenfell, B. T., Pybus, O. G., & Dye, C. (2020). An investigation of transmission control measures during the first 50 days of the COVID-19 epidemic in China. *Science*, 368(6491): 638–642. doi:10.1126/science.abb6105

Tomova, L., Wang, K. L., Thompson, T., Matthews, G. A., Takahashi, A., Tye, K. M., & Saxe, R. (2020). Acute social isolation evokes midbrain craving responses similar to hunger. *Nature Neuroscience*, 23: 1597–1605.

Walsh, C. (2021, 17th February). Young adults hardest hit by loneliness during pandemic. *The Harvard Gazette*. Retrieved from: https://news.harvard.edu/gazette/story/2021/02/young-adults-teens-loneliness-mental-health-coronavirus-covid-pandemic/

Wang, J., Mann. F., Lloyd-Evans, B., Ma R., & Johnson, S. (2018 May 29). Associations between loneliness and perceived social support and outcomes of mental health problems: A systematic review. *BMC Psychiatry*, 18(1): 156. doi: 10.1186/s12888-018-1736-5

Wang, H. X., Mittleman, M. A., & Orth-Gomer, K. (2005). Influence of social support on progression of coronary artery disease in women. *Social Science and Medicine*, 60: 599–607.

Warttig, S. L., Forshaw, M. J., South, J., & White, A. K. (2013). New, normative, English-sample data for the Short Form Perceived Stress Scale (PSS-4). *Journal of Health Psychology*, 18(12): 1617–1628. doi: 10.1177/1359105313508346

Williams, S. N., Armitage, C. J., Tampe, T., et al. (2020). Public perceptions and experiences of social distancing and social isolation during the COVID-19 pandemic: A UK-based focus group study. *BMJ Open*, 10: e039334.

Williams, W. C., Morelli, S. A., Ong, D. C. & Zaki, J. (2018). Interpersonal emotion regulation: Implications for affiliation, perceived support, relationships, and well-being. *Journal of Personality and Social Psychology*, 115: 224–254.

Willeumier, K. (2021, 21st February). How social isolation and loneliness impact brain function. *Psychology Today*. https://www.psychologytoday.com/us/blog/biohack-your-brain/202102/how-social-isolation-and-loneliness-impact-brain-function

Worsley, R., & Williams, R. (2020, 16th April). COVID-19 and mental well-being. Ipsos-MORI. Available at: https://www.ipsos.com/ipsos-mori/en-uk/Covid-19-and-mental-wellbeing

YouGov (2020, 9th October). What impact would you say that the coronavirus pandemic has had, if at all, on your mental health. Available at: https://yougov.co.uk/topics/health/survey-results/daily/2020/10/09/26286/2

YouGov (2020, 9th October). How often, if at all, have you felt lonely in the last two months? Available at: https://yougov.co.uk/topics/health/survey-results/daily/2020/10/09/26286/3

Yu, G., Renton, A., Wall, M., Estacio, E., Cawley, J., & Datta P. (2011). Prevalence of low physical activity and its relation to social environment in deprived areas in the London Borough of Redbridge. *Social Indicators Research*, 104(2): 311–322.

Zhang, S. X., Wang, Y., Rauch, A., & Wei, F. (2020). Unprecedented Disruption of lives and work: Health, distress, and life satisfaction of working adults in china one month into the COVID-19 Outbreak.*Psychiatry Research*, 288(112958): 1–6.

Zhou, F., Yu, T., Du, R., Fan, G., Liu, Y., Liu, Z., Xiang, J., Wang, Y., Song, B., Gu, X., Guan, L., Wei, Y., Li, H., Wu, X., Xu, J., Tu, S., Zhang, Y., Chen, H., & Cao B. (2020). Clinical course and risk factors for mortality of adult inpatients with COVID-19 in Wuhan, China: A retrospective cohort study. *Lancet*, 395(10229): 1054–1062. doi: 10.1016/S0140-6736(20)30566-3

Chapter 4

Lockdown and Mental Health

Historically, research into the psychological impacts of epidemics had shown that when authorities imposed severe restrictions on public behaviour, this could seriously influence the psychological health of those affected. Much of the earlier evidence had relied on cross-sectional surveys that examined relationships between severity of behavioural restrictions, concerns about new diseases and status of psychological health at one point in time (Brooks et al., 2020). Much more could be learned about the effects of pandemics by studying how people respond to them over time. In other words, it is important to know whether there are measurable changes in the psychological health of people during a pandemic as compared with how they were before it.

Evidence emerged during the novel coronavirus pandemic that psychological health could be adversely affected by the new pandemic (de Quervain et al., 2020; Wang et al., 2020). This confirmed research into the way people reacted in countries previously affected by coronaviruses, such as in the 2002–2003 SARS (severe acute respiratory syndrome) outbreak in the Far East and the 2012 MERS (Middle East respiratory syndrome) outbreak in the Middle East which indicated that pandemics, even when not worldwide, can cause mental health problems for those affected. Social isolation and quarantining measures were taken by national governments to combat these two diseases and provide test models for coping with the 2020 pandemic.

Earlier research had covered child and adult populations from China, Hong Kong, Japan, South Korea, Saudi Arabia, France, the United Kingdom, Canada and the United States (Rogers et al., 2020). This evidence is derived from people followed-up within a matter of months of a pandemic outbreak or many years afterwards. Individuals infected by these diseases, that had sometimes necessitated admittance to hospital, often suffered from anxiety, depression, insomnia and other cognitive functioning problems. These symptoms were not only experienced during illness but subsequently persisted for some time after recovery. Some patients

DOI: 10.4324/9781003274377-4

experienced more severe symptoms such as delirium and post-traumatic stress disorders (PTSD).

The Mental Health Foundation tracked the status of people's mental health in the United Kingdom during the pandemic through its *Coronavirus: Mental Health in the Pandemic* study (Mental Health Foundation, 2020). Its research found that even though the government's measures during the pandemic were well-intentioned, they provided better protection for some groups in society than for others. Short-term and longer-term consequences of the lockdown meant that some people suffered from significant changes to their lifestyles that did nothing to improve their overall state of well-being and many people experienced mental health issues. Even people that ordinarily did not experience anxiety or depression began to do so during the lockdown, but those already suffering from mental health problems often found that their overall condition deteriorated.

Anxiety, Distress and the Threat of Infection

For many people, their initial anxiety responses were linked to their fear of infection. There were also anxiety responses linked to governments' restrictions on public behaviour, in part, because these underlined the seriousness of the situation and also because, for many people, their livelihoods were put under threat and they were prevented from seeing close family members they were worried about.

Online research carried out with 56,000 people across China during the early phase of the pandemic (28th February to 11th March 2020) with adults (aged 18+) found that anxiety (32%), depression (28%), insomnia (29%) and acute stress symptoms (24%) were widely reported. These symptoms tended to be more prevalent among individuals who suspected they or members of their family had had COVID-19. Another factor that enhanced negative mental health reactions to the pandemic such as anxiety and depression was the extent to which their job put them at greater risk of infection. Being back at work, however, seemed to give some protection against anxiety, depression and insomnia, while being quarantined triggered anxiety responses and increased reports of depression (Shi et al., 2020).

Soundings that were taken of mental health responses among young people in low- and middle-income developing countries such as Ethiopia, India, Peru and Vietnam showed that the prevalence of mild pandemic-related anxiety varied between a low of 9% in Vietnam to a high of 41% in Peru (Porter et al., 2020).

Catching COVID-19 could have a real impact, psychologically, on those infected, but for most people this was short-lived. The level of worry in this context might depend also on how seriously ill those infected became. A study of 8,000+ Americans, from April 2020 to February 2021 showed that psychological distress was triggered by COVID-19. This was elevated for around two weeks after respondents were first tested positive, remained elevated for a further two weeks, before then settling down closer to pre-infection levels. Psychological distress was most severe among those who became more seriously ill with COVID-19. The initial diagnosis was a stressor for many people. Then experiencing symptoms could add to this or not depending upon how serious they became (Daly & Robinson, 2021).

Research from Japan found that one in three people reported mild to moderate distress, (37%) and over one in ten (12%) reported more serious levels of distress, as measured by clinically validated psychological tests during COVID-19 lockdown. The proportions of people that reported experiencing psychological stress was significantly higher than comparable national data for 2010, 2013, 2016 and 2019. Healthcare workers, those with a history of mental illness and adults aged under 40, were especially likely to have suffered adverse psychological side-effects. Other psychological factors such as loneliness, poor interpersonal relationships and disrupted sleep patterns as well as loss of income and future employment threats were also related to higher levels of reported distress (Yamamoto et al., 2020). A study covering Argentina and China found that chronic anxiety could develop from persistent fears about getting infected. For some people, this could then translate into depression symptoms (for some Fernández, Crivelli, Guimet, Allegri, & Pedreira, 2020; Zhang et al., 2020).

Anxiety Responses to Lockdown

From early in the pandemic, behavioural scientists believed that social distancing measures contributed towards the emergence of mental disorders during the pandemic as individuals were starved of normal human-to-human contact. For some people, the practice of social distancing made them feel more in control and this decreased the severity of adverse psychological side-effects. For others, however, the opposite was true – social distancing felt isolating and this gave rise to its own psychological problems. Pre-existing status of mental health also played into this process and rendered some people more vulnerable and at risk than others from the start (Van Rheene et al., 2020).

Evidence from across China found that over half of the samples surveyed (54%) said that the pandemic had had a moderate to the severe psychological impact on them. A minority (17%) reported increased depression. The great majority of these people (85%) hardly ever left their home over many weeks and most (75%) were worried about family members contracting the virus (Wang et al., 2020). Those with other health conditions tended to be more anxious about getting the new virus. Where coping mechanisms were available and could be adopted by people, such as wearing face masks and being diligent about hand hygiene, the registered psychological impact (e.g., feeling anxious, stressed or depressed) was lessened (Wang et al., 2020).

A study of college students in China found a presence of acute stress (35%), depression (21%) and anxiety (11%) during the pandemic. Having relatives and friends that had been infected by COVID-19 enhanced the risk of mental health problems during the pandemic. Having had greater exposure to media coverage of the pandemic also aggravated these mental health side-effects. When students said they had plenty of social support, they were less likely to experience anxiety and depressive symptoms (Ma et al., 2020).

In the Czech Republic, people reported increased experience of psychological symptoms such as poor mood state, anxiety, depression and suicidal thoughts during the pandemic. Anxiety was especially likely to have increased at this time. There was further evidence of increased alcohol abuse in the form of binge drinking. These reactions were also associated with how much respondents worried about their financial circumstances and their health (Winkler et al., 2020).

Further research from Saudi Arabia found that nearly one in four people (24%) surveyed said they had experienced moderate or severe psychological symptoms during the pandemic and specific symptoms included reports of depression (28%) anxiety (24%) and stress (22%). Such reports were more prevalent among women than men and were more widespread among high-school students, those working in the medical field, and those who said they had generally poorer health. Practising specific preventative measures such as hand-washing and social distancing was associated with more modest levels of adverse psychological reactions (Alkhamees et al., 2020).

In the United Kingdom, low tolerance of lockdown and the uncertainty it created could trigger anxiety responses in many people. In an online survey conducted during 10 days the early phase of the first lockdown in the United Kingdom, researchers found elevated anxiety levels. This response was especially prevalent among people who were already anxious about their health (Rettie & Daniels, 2020).

The COVID-19 Psychological Research Consortium (C19PRC) followed through the impact of the pandemic on the public's behaviour in the United Kingdom across the March to July 2020 period of the pandemic. This research covered only an early phase of the period of pandemic-related behavioural restrictions which in the United Kingdom lasted for another year. Nevertheless, with survey waves conducted in March, April and July 2020, it did provide early longitudinal insights of developing mental health issues from which longer-term effects might emerge. In one specific study that focused on mental health effects, the researchers measured reported occurrences of anxiety, depression and PTSD using established psychological tests. In general, the prevalence of anxiety and depression was fairly stable across this period of observation. The incidence of reported PTSD symptoms decreased from April to July 2020. Some people therefore seemed to develop psychological coping mechanisms from early on. Others did not. In all, nearly one in three (around 30%) exhibited rising anxiety and depression symptoms (Shevlin et al., 2021).

Other studies were conducted during this period that were already running before the pandemic struck and draconian behavioural restrictions had been put in place. This allowed for pre-pandemic benchmarks with which to compare pandemic reactions. One such study was carried out in the United Kingdom and another in the US offering an international comparison. In the United Kingdom, the prevalence of reported distress among adults surveyed increased notably from the pre-pandemic sounding (19%) to another take during the first month of the first national lockdown in April 2020 (27%) (Pierce et al., 2020). An American study noted a similar margin of change on this variable from before the pandemic (4%) in 2018 to after it in April 2020 (14%) (McGinty et al., 2020b). Some notes of caution were advised with these studies.

Although their population sampling procedures were robust, their measures of people's psychological state were less so. Furthermore, while the pre-pandemic surveys in both studies were conducted through face-to-face interviews, because of COVID-19 restrictions the researchers had to switch to web-based surveys during the pandemic (see Burton et al., 2020; McGinty et al., 2020b; Pierce et al., 2020). The US study was also methodologically blighted by the fact that different parts of the country introduced pandemic-related restrictions at different times and did not invariably impose the same restrictions.

During the pandemic, another longitudinal exercise from the United States found little change in the proportion of people saying they had experienced serious psychological distress (14–13%) during the early pandemic (McGinty et al., 2020a). Between March and May 2020 in Ireland, anxiety reports (20% and 17%) and symptomatic depression reports (23% and 24%) also exhibited small or marginal changes in reporting levels over time (Hyland et al., 2021). These findings were repeated in the United Kingdom with reportedly decreased rates of anxiety and no change in depression (O'Connor et al., 2020). Other British research found modest but decreased rates of reporting of both anxiety and depression (Fancourt et al., 2021).

In general, research from different countries conducted during the early phases of the pandemic, that is, through spring and summer of 2020, indicated that people were initially made anxious by the pandemic experience and some even became depressed. These responses, however, stabilised over time. This pattern of responding is consistent with the explanation that when people are placed under stress many of them will work out ways of coping with it. It is important to note in the case of British studies especially that by July 2020, the United Kingdom government increasingly put out messages about lifting pandemic restrictions. Indeed, by that time some restrictions had already been lifted. This gave many people a sense of hope that the worst was over (YouGov, 2020a).

Early data indicated that while many people exhibited resilience in the face of the crisis, no one knew how long this resilience would last if they were confronted with repeat waves of society being closed down. Prior research had indicated that populations bounce back after major national disasters and crises but those observations were made for events that did not keep recurring (Bonanno, 2004; Goldmann and Galea, 2014).

Gender and Pandemic-Related Psychological Impact

There was evidence that women often reported feeling the strain more so than did men. Whether this was because they really were more stressed by pandemic interventions or were simply more likely to admit to feeling this way than were men is not always easy to disentangle. There were other experiential factors in play here as well. Women were less likely than men to die from COVID-19, but in many ways they had found the pandemic experience harder to cope with mentally. Women were more likely to have stayed home from work where they were confronted with domestic as well as work pressures. Women felt more pressure to take care of their family who were also at home (Hamel & Salganikoff, 2020). Women were more likely than men to have been laid off from their jobs at least temporarily with all financial pressures that could bring. Over a series of polls conducted between March 2020 and April 2021, data had shown a consistently higher prevalence of loneliness and anxiety among women than among men (Office of National Statistics, 2021, 10th March).

French research showed that being female or nonbinary, combined with having a precarious income, living in poor quality housing, having a history of psychiatric symptoms, having experienced COVID-19 symptoms, being socially isolated, having poor social relations anyway and having received only poor-quality information about COVID-19 were all risk factors that enhanced the likelihood of experiencing serious psychological symptoms (Wathelet et al., 2020).

One dynamic at play was that women generally had wider and more regularly supportive social networks than did men. Being prohibited from direct contact with these often meant that women experienced these enforced social and psychological deprivation conditions more deeply than did men. The latter reaction was evidenced in more widespread reports of loneliness from women than from men during the early phases of pandemic-related restrictions (Chandola et al., 2020; Fancourt et al., 2020; Jia et al., 2020; Xue & McMunn, 2020; Ellwardt & Präg, 2021).

Other evidence emerged from Italy that women were more likely than men to report mental health deterioration and, in particular, to feel generally more anxious and depressed. Further, knowing someone who had become infected by the virus was also associated with greater reported stress and depression, especially if this was a family member (Mazza et al., 2020). In Israel, women tended to be more susceptible to anxiety reactions than were men especially if they had pre-existing health problems (Horesh et al., 2020). In Iran, in contrast, no significant differences in reports of COVID anxiety and depression were found between women and men (Mohammadpour et al., 2020).

Other conditions and circumstances could also come into play to mitigate against worsening unpleasant symptoms of pandemic lockdowns and other restrictions. Pregnant women were found to voice louder concern about the anxiety and distress the pandemic had caused them (Talbot et al., 2020). In different parts of the world, for example, they were found to voice louder concern about the anxiety and distress the pandemic had caused them (Ostacoli et al., 2020; Talbot et al., 2020).

In China, exposure to COVID-related information registered more profound and negative psychological impacts on women than on men (Hou et al., 2020). In Canada, women students reported more stress and mental health symptoms than did men. These women were also more likely to turn to social media as a distraction although this was also found to contribute further to their anxiety symptoms because of the COVID-related content they found there (Prowse et al., 2021). In Spain, women from 18 to 84 exhibited more severe anxiety and stress reactions to COVID-19 and the pandemic than did men (García-Fernández et al., 2020).

Personality and COVID-19 Anxiety

Differences in anxiety responses to the pandemic could in part be explained by personality differences between people. These psychological factors represent defining characteristics of a person which determine to a great extent how they will behave in different settings. Personality was found to relate also to anxiety responses to the pandemic. In different parts of the world, from China to North America, people with pre-existing mental health vulnerabilities exhibited the most severe negative responses as the pandemic got underway. Those with stronger personalities protected by their inherent optimism and self-sufficiency fared much better (Asmundson et al., 2020; Song et al., 2021).

One of the most widely used models of personality has become known as the "Big Five". In reminding ourselves about this model, it comprises five personality dimensions popularly labelled as Agreeableness, Conscientiousness, Extraversion, Neuroticism and Openness to Experience (McCrae & Costa, 1987; Goldberg, 1993). This model was used in pandemic-related studies of psychological reactions to COVID-19 and related interventions. In Spain, individuals who scored low on Neuroticism and high on Agreeableness, Conscientiousness and Extraversion generally exhibited better mental health, especially in terms of anxiety scores during the pandemic (López-Núñez et al., 2020). These results were replicated in the United States where it also emerged that higher Openness to Experience was linked to developing chronic anxiety (Nikcevic et al., 2020). The risk of higher Neuroticism to adverse anxiety responses during the pandemic was further observed in India (Pradhan et al., 2020; Somma et al., 2020).

Other personality factors were found to promote anxiety responses during the pandemic. Lower scorers on dimensions such as psychological flexibility and uncertainty tolerance exhibited reduced well-being and greater anxiety during the pandemic (Pakenham et al., 2020; Ran et al., 2020; Wielgus et al., 2020). People who were more uncomfortable with uncertain situations were more prone to experience anxiety during the pandemic (Rettie & Daniels, 2020).

Interventions and Anxiety Responses

As well as the disease itself, there were further anxieties triggered by the interventions imposed by authorities that caused economic and psychological strains coupled with uncertainties over how long these new restrictive conditions would last for. Under these conditions, people can often find it difficult to concentrate on their everyday lives, and this reaction can undermine their ability to focus on their work, whether they were still travelling into their normal workplace or were working from home. There were then systemic anxieties about the ability of their country's health services to cope with the crisis situation with which they were confronted (Kestilä et al., 2020; Trougakos et al., 2020; Waizenegger et al., 2020).

Welcomed by some, for many others, being forced to work from home was associated with the loss of the social contact of work where individuals would enjoy mixing with other colleagues at the office. The absence of that contact might create a sense of social isolation that could in turn lead to anxiety or depression responses (Charoensukmongkol & Phungsoonthorn, 2020; Evanoff et al., 2020). This isolation and lack of a sense of support could become even more pronounced when employers had not thought through how these basic needs might be satisfied under these dramatically changed working conditions (Charoensukmongkol & Phungsoonthorn, 2020; Evanoff et al., 2020) Employees that felt abandoned once confined to working from home, especially where their employer had failed to develop new methods of retaining team cohesion in remote working settings, could quickly develop chronic anxiety symptoms (Ruiz-Frutos et al., 2021).

Social Isolation, Uncertainty and Anxiety

The uncertainty created by the COVID-19 pandemic could trigger a range of psychological reactions, many of which were not healthy. Most common among the responses were anxiety and panic (see Chapter 6 for discussion of panic buying). These feelings could not only motivate people to behave in unusual ways (e.g., panic buying of commodities in the belief that they might be in short supply if many people are off work sick with the new virus or that they themselves might not be able to shop for essentials if they get ill, loss of sleep, loss of appetite (or comfort eating), digestive upsets and other more extreme stress symptoms (Rogers et al., 2020).

Although uncertainty in the face of a situation that presents a risk to the individual can provoke anxiety on its own, the presence of social isolation can create a potentially more chronic type of response that causes longer-lasting harm resulting from the lack of interaction with other people (Leigh-Hunt et al., 2017). Research conducted during the pandemic found that even relatively short periods of social isolation or no more than 10 days at a time can have lasting effects (Brooks et al., 2020). Prolonged social isolation can have even more damaging effects. These can include not just feeling anxious or depressed, but more fundamental influences such as impaired cognitive functioning and physical health effects aggravated by a compromised immune *system* (Cohen et al., 1997; Barth et al., 2010; Heffner et al., 2011).

Social isolation can also interact with loneliness to damage a person's sense of well-being and their actual health. It does not invariably follow that social isolation results in feelings of loneliness. Being alone and being lonely are not the same. Moreover, a person can feel "lonely" even though they have regular social contact with others. In this case, how an individual labels their current state (i.e., as "being lonely") can depend upon the nature and quality of relationships they have with others. Nonetheless, being required or forced to isolate from others can exacerbate the feelings of those who already report being lonely (Shankar et al., 2011).

Loneliness is not simply a commonly used term for a personal feeling or behavioural state, it is now identified as a clinical condition that influences health (Grant et al., 2009; Cole et al., 2015: Bzdok & Dunbar, 2020). One established it is a condition that can persist and then becomes a risk factor in relation to mental health (Cacioppo et al., 2006; Han & Richardson, 2010; Hawker & Romero-Ortuno, 2016).

Loneliness and Psychological State

Another factor at play, which cut across demographics and occupations, was loneliness (YouGov, 2020b). The implementation of social distancing, social isolation and quarantining interventions meant that many people were starved of social contact. Attention often focused on those people – often the elderly – that were already socially disconnected, but it could be those who were normally socially very active that suffered the most under these socially restrictive conditions because they had not developed coping mechanisms for living alone. "Loneliness" is not so much a physical state defined by whether a person lives on their own, but rather it is a psychological state underpinned by the way individuals perceive themselves and their lives. The self-perception of being not so much "alone", but "lonely", was connected to an increased risk of anxiety reactions to the pandemic (Gaeta & Brydges, 2020; Xu et al., 2020).

Despite the necessity of quarantining and social isolation interventions to deal with the spread of a mostly airborne novel coronavirus, studies from different parts of the world showed that up to one-fifth of people affected by these measures experienced some degree of psychological distress. This often took the form of generalised anxiety but could also develop into more serious symptoms such as depression and PTSD (Cavicchioli et al., 2021).

Using the Spielberger State-Trait Anxiety Inventory, Finnish researchers found evidence of COVID-related anxiety that was influenced by loneliness, distress and social isolation, both from friends and work colleagues, and by the concept of "technostress" which stemmed from working remotely at home which often led to work for much longer hours. Work from home also created tensions for some people because the usual clear divide between work life and home life had been eroded under these exceptional circumstances. Individuals who scored high on the neuroticism personality trait also reported greater COVID-related anxiety symptoms (Savolainen et al., 2021).

Sleep Disturbances

One psychological outcome of the lockdown was an interesting change to people's sleep experiences. Sleep, and especially dream sleep, is important for good mental and physical health. When sleep is disturbed, often through stress, dreaming can also be disrupted. Many of us forget our dreams because we do not wake up before they have ended. If we do, and the dream has not completed its cycle, we are more likely to recall what we were dreaming about. If we repeatedly awaken during the night, a phenomenon known as a parasomnia – and exhibit increased dream recall, this is a signal that we are not sleeping effectively (Renner, 2020).

One study in France, during the COVID-19 lockdown, found that the pandemic had caused a 35% increase in dream recall. Not only that, but some people (around 15%) reported experiencing more unpleasant dreams. Similar findings were reported by research in Italy (Renner, 2020). In a United Kingdom survey conducted by King's College London and Ipsos-MORI in May 2020, two in five people reported experiencing strange dreams during the COVID-19 lockdown. Further evidence showed that respondents that reported feeling under stress were the most likely to say they had had such dreams. Anecdotally, other evidence started to accumulate that people reported having very vivid dreams about the lockdown, post-lockdown parties and work-related matters. This phenomenon was not restricted to people in Britain.

Reports came back from people in the United States about having unusual lockdown dreams. Experts noted that there was mounting evidence that many people, perhaps as many as one in two, were experiencing disturbed sleep during the lockdown period. Often, this phenomenon is accompanied by waking up before the end of a dream. This means that usually the dream remains unfinished or unresolved, but also it tends to be remembered. When dreams can complete their cycle without the dreamer waking up, they tend not to be remembered. Hence, more dream reports could have signalled that people were more anxious and this was disrupting their normal sleep pattern (Crisell, 2020).

With the pandemic over a year old in the United Kingdom, few people (8%) reported that they were getting very good quality sleep. This finding revealed a significant deterioration (by 39%) since the start of the pandemic. Improved sleep quality over the year was found among older adults, those without mental health conditions, men (rather than women), those of white ethnicity and people not living with children. The overall proportion reporting very poor sleep increased from just over 5% in the autumn 2020 to just over 10% in early 2021 (Fancourt et al., 2021).

Getting COVID and Cognitive Impairment

"Brain fog" is not a medical term but it has been used to represent symptoms reported by individuals who claim to have experienced difficulties with their attention and cognitive functioning after having been infected by COVID-19. It was known that COVID-19 sufferers could sometimes experience longer-term debilitating or unpleasant symptoms collectively subsumed under the generic heading of "long COVID" (Budson, 2021).

Similar symptoms were reported as reactions to the general pressures and stress many people experienced during the pandemic (White, 2020). These are derived not just from being infected by the new virus but also by the associated extreme behavioural restrictions imposed upon people by their governments. Uncertainty created by widespread closure of societies for unknown time durations triggered collective stress and chronic anxiety across entire populations.

While it was known that COVID-19 could cause respiratory problems, mounting evidence also indicated that neurological systems could also be adversely impacted. One American study found that 42% of people displayed neurological symptoms soon after catching the virus, increasing to 63% among those admitted to hospital and 82% overall at some point during infection (Liotta et al., 2020).

Neurological problems can occur if the infection results in poor oxygen supply to the brain which leads in turn to psychological changes that undermine normal cognitive functioning and behaviour. The hippocampus seems to be especially susceptible to coronavirus infections and this is a primary site for orchestrating memory functioning and performance (Ritchie et al., 2020).

The Great British Intelligence Test was designed to understand cognitive ability distribution across the population and how it might be affected by a range of personal and experiential factors in people's lives. It was launched in January 2020 and data were collected on a regular basis throughout the remainder of the year. In all, more than 81,000 people took part. In the May 2020 survey questions were included about COVID-19. Nearly 13,000 people reported mild to severe symptoms known to be associated with COVID-19. Matching people by age and education, findings showed that those that had apparently caught COVID-19 and been hospitalised subsequently displayed poorer cognitive function, especially on skills such as problem-solving, reasoning and spatial planning than did others uninfected or less seriously ill with the new disease. For some, cognitive decline was highly significant and similar in scale to 10 years of ageing-related decline (Hampshire et al., 2021).

This work was supported by research conducted with COVID-related hospitalised patients that reported impaired cognitive functioning and for whom further observations revealed that they had diminished capacities to look after themselves and perform simple cognitive and behavioural tasks even many months after release from hospital (Frontera et al., 2021).

Lessons Learned

One of the most far-reaching collateral side-effects of the pandemic and governments' interventions around the world was greater amounts of public anxiety. For some people, there were understandable fear responses to the pandemic, especially during its early stages when the seriousness of the disease was not yet understood. Yet, the decisions by most governments effectively to shut down their economies and societies, an unprecedented experience for virtually everyone on the planet, underlined to people that the situation was serious.

With the disease being established as airborne and highly infectious, and with no vaccines or established drug therapies available, governments turned to non-pharmaceutical interventions that became manifest as extreme behaviour control measures. The principal objective was to keep people apart from others as much as possible to prevent one from infecting another. This enforced socially isolation broke down social support networks and starved many people of social contact to a point that the interventions themselves became as big a source of potential harm to public health as the new virus.

In this chapter, research has been examined from around the world that investigated the mental health effects of the pandemic. As noted, this showed that public anxiety levels became higher than usual, but these heightened psychological reactions did not always persist. Over time, it seems, many people, wherever in the world they were, managed to get their initial anxiety symptoms under control. This coping phenomenon was not achieved by everyone. People prone to be anxious anyway, because of their personality type, were still anxious and stayed that way. There were others who became chronically anxious because of the effects of the pandemic and who experienced stress as well. These reactions were especially likely to occur among people most seriously affected by the pandemic because it changed their work routines or their domestic routines, of threatened their jobs or resulted in job loss and the accompanying financial worries that went with that.

Then there were people who knew someone who had died of COVID-19 who had good reason to be threatened by it. There were people who worked on the frontline in health and social care who continued to go to work and where their workplace confronted them everyday with a real risk of infection (Alshekai et al., 2020; Huang et al., 2020; Liang et al., 2020).

A broad overview, historically, of the psychological impact of epidemics or pandemics on healthcare workers was provided in a review of 44 studies that had investigated anxiety, depression, post-traumatic stress and general psychiatric symptoms reported by doctors, nurses and auxiliary staff on these occasions (Preti et al., 2020). Results varied widely from one study to another and from epidemic/pandemic to another. Post-traumatic stress was reported by between 11% and 73% of healthcare workers during these outbreaks. Depression was reported by 28–51%. Insomnia was reported by 34–36%. Severe anxiety symptoms were reported by 45%. General psychiatric problems ranged widely from 17% to 75%. These responses could be aggravated by greater levels of exposure to infected patients, degree of organisation support during these crises and, in particular, by the adequacy of provision of protective equipment.

Other research revealed that persistent anxiety and stress could, for some people evolved into depression (Planchuelo-Gómez et al., 2020; Wang et al., 2020). As research from Italy found, some people got stressed or depressed at the start of the pandemic and stayed that way. Those most prone to experience pandemic stress and depression were people with fewer conditioned coping mechanisms for managing these reactions from their earlier life (Roma et al., 2020).

For some people, sleep was also disturbed during the pandemic. There was evidence not only that the amount of sleep was affected, but also the quality of sleep. This was measured in terms of dream sleep. There were increased reports by people of having strange dreams or dreams from which they awoke prematurely meaning that they were never resolved.

In general, then, it appears there was widespread collateral mental health damage caused by the pandemic and by the effects of pandemic-related interventions. Some people reacted severely to the threat of the new disease. Others felt under pressure when their usual social support systems were taken away from them. Loneliness grew and sowed the psychological seeds for internal responses that could be serious for those already vulnerable to anxiety and depression. Going forward, it will be important to establish the longer-lasting effects of the pandemic experience. Despite signs that some anxious people managed to get their negative feelings under control during the early stages of the pandemic, many were perhaps reassured by a mistaken belief that the pandemic would soon be over. The reality was, for many, that it went on for much longer than they anticipated allowing more time for severe psychological side-effects to become embedded.

References

Ahrens, K. F., Neumann, R. J., Kollmann, B., Plichta, M. M., Lieb, K., Tüscher, O., & Reif, A. (2021). Differential impact of COVID-related lockdown on mental health in Germany. *World Psychiatry*, 20(1): 140–141. doi: 10.1002/wps.20830

Alkhamees, A. A., Alrashed, S. A., Alzunaydi, A. A., Almohimeed, A. S., & Aljohani, M. S. (2020). The psychological impact of COVID-19 pandemic on the general population of Saudi Arabia. *Comparative Psychiatry*, 102: 152192. doi: 10.1016/j.comppsych.2020.152192

Alshekai, M., Hassan, W., Al Said, N., Al Sulaimani, F., Jayapal, S. K., Al-Mawali, A., Chan, M. F., Mahadevan, S., & Al-Adawi, S. (2020). Factors associated with mental health outcomes across healthcare settings in Oman during COVID-19: Frontline versus non-frontline healthcare workers. *BMJ Open*, 10(10): e042030. doi: 10.1136/bmjopen-2020-042030

Asmundson, G. J. G., Paluszek, M. M., Landry, C. A., Rachor, G. S., McKay, D., & Taylor, S. (2020). Do pre-existing anxiety-related and mood disorders differentially impact COVID-19 stress responses and coping? *Journal of Anxiety Disorders*, 74: 102271. doi: 10.1016/j.janxdis.2020.102271

Asparouhov, T., & Muthén, B. (2014). Auxiliary variables in mixture modeling: Using the BCH method in Mplus to estimate a distal outcome model and an arbitrary secondary model. *Mplus Web Notes*, 21(2): 1–22.

Barth, J. S., Schneider, S., & von Känel, R. (2010). Lack of social support in the etiology and the prognosis of coronary heart disease: A systematic review and meta-analysis. *Psychosomatic Medicine*, 72: 229–238. doi: 10.1097/PSY.0b013e3181d01611

Bauer, D. J., & Curran, P. J. (2003). Distributional assumptions of growth mixture models: Implications for over-extraction of latent classes. *Psychological Methods*, 8: 338–363. doi: 10.1037/1082-989X.8.3.338

Ben-Ezra, M., Karatzias, T., Hyland, P., Brewin, C. R., Cloitre, M., Bisson, J. I., Roberts, N. P., Lueger-Schuster, B., & Shevlin, M. (2018). Posttraumatic stress disorder (PTSD) and complex PTSD (CPTSD) as per ICD-11 proposals: A population study in Israel. *Depression and Anxiety*, 35(3): 264–274. doi: 10.1002/da.22723

Bonanno, G. A. (2004). Loss, trauma, and human resilience: Have we under-estimated the human capacity to thrive after extremely aversive events? *American Psychologist*, 59(1): 20–28. doi: 10.1037/0003-066X.59.1.20

Brooks, S. K., Webster, R. K., Smith, L. E., Woodland, L., Wessely, S., Greenberg, N., & Rubin, J. G. (2020). The psychological impact of quarantine and how to reduce it: Rapid review of the evidence. *The Lancet*, 395(10227): 912–920.

Budson, A. E. (2021, 8th March). What is COVID-19 brain fog – and how can you clear it? Harvard health Blog, Harvard Medical School. Retrieved from: https://www.health.harvard.edu/blog/what-is-covid-19-brain-fog-and-how-can-you-clear-it-2021030822076

Burton, J., Lynn, P., & Benzeval, M. (2020). How understanding society: The UK household longitudinal study adapted to the COVID-19 pandemic. *Survey Research Methods*, 14(2): 235–239. doi: 10.18148/srm/2020.v14i2.7746

Bzdok, D., & Dunbar, R. I. M. (2020). The neurobiology of social distance. *Trends in Cognitive Sciences*, 24(9): 717–733. doi: 10.1016/j.tics.2020.05.016

Cacioppo, J. T., Hughes, M. E., Waite, L. J., Hawkley, L. C., & Thisted, R. A. (2006). Loneliness as a specific risk factor for depressive symptoms: Cross-sectional and longitudinal analyses. *Psychology of Aging*, 21(1): 140–151.

Cavicchioli, M., Ferrucci, R., Guidetti, M., Cancuini, M. P., Pravettoni, G., & Gali, F. (2021). From Covid-19 to psychological distress: A systematic review on quarantine. *Healthcare*, 9: 101. https://www.preprints.org/manuscript/202012.0135/v1

Chandola, T., Kumari, M., Booker, C. L., & Benzeval, M. J. (2020). The mental health impact of COVID-19 and pandemic related stressors among adults in the UK. *Psychological Medicine*, 1–10. doi: 10.1017/S0033291720005048

Charoensukmongkol, P., & Phungsoonthorn, T. (2020). The effectiveness of su-pervisor support in lessening perceived uncertainties and emotional exhaustion of university employees during the COVID-19 crisis: The constraining role of or-ganizational intransigence. *Journal of General Psychology*, 148(4): 269–286. doi: 10.1080/00221309.2020.1795613

Chauvenet, A., Buckley, R., Hague, L., Fleming, C., & Brough, P. (2020). Panel sampling in health research. The Lancet Psychiatry, 7(10): 840–841. doi: 10.1016/S2215-0366(20)30358-8

Cohen, S., Doyle, W. J., Skoner, D. P., Rabin, B. S., & Gwaltney, J. M. Jr. (1997). Social ties and susceptibility to the common cold. *JAMA*, 277: 1940–1944. doi: 10.1001/jama.1997.03540480040036

Cole, S. W., Capitanio, J. P., Chun, K., Arevalo, J. M., Ma, J., & Cacioppo, J. T. (2015). Myeloid differentiation architecture of leukocyte transcriptome dynamics in perceived social isolation. *Proceedings of the National Academy of Science of the USA*, 112, 15142–15147. doi: 10.1073/pnas.1514249112

Crisell, H. (2020, 8th June). Covid dreams: How strange are yours? *The Times: Times 2*, pp. 2–3.

Daly, M., & Robinson, E. (2021). Acute and longer-term psychological distress associated with testing positive for COVID-19: longitudinal evidence from a population-based study of US adults. *Journal of Psychiatric Research*, 136: 603–609. https://doi.org/10.1016/j.jpsychires.2020.10.035

De Quervain, D., Aerni, A., Amini, E., Bentz, D., Coynel, D., Gerhards, C., … Zuber, P. (2020). The Swiss Corona stress study. [Preprint]. Retrieved from https://osf.io/jqw6a

Diallo, T. M. O., Morin, A. J. S., & Lu, H. (2016). Impact of misspecifications of the latent variance–covariance and residual matrices on the class enumeration accuracy of growth mixture models. *Structural Equation Modeling*, 23(4): 507–531. doi: 10.1080/10705511.2016.1169188

Ellwardt, L., & Präg, P. (2021). Heterogeneous mental health development during the COVID-19 pandemic in the United Kingdom. *Science Reports*, 11(1): 15958. doi: 10.1038/s41598-021-95490-w

Evanoff, B. A., Strickland, J. R., Dale, A. M., Hayibor, L., Page, E., Duncan, J. G., & Gray, D. L. (2020). Work-related and personal factors associated with mental well-being during COVID-19 Response: A survey of health care and other workers. *Journal of Medicine and Internet Research*, 22: e21366.

Fancourt, D., Steptoe, A., & Bu, F. (2021). Trajectories of anxiety and depressive symptoms during enforced isolation due to COVID-19 in England: A longitudinal observational study. *The Lancet Psychiatry*, 8(2): 141–149. 10.1016/S2215-0366(20)30482-X

Fang, X., Zhang, J., Teng, C., Zhao, K., Su, K.-P., Wang, Z., Tang, W., & Zhang, C. (2020). Depressive symptoms in the front-line non-medical workers during the COVID-19 outbreak in Wuhan. *Journal of Affective Disorders*, 276: 441–445.

Fernández, R. S., Crivelli, L., Guimet, N. M., Allegri, R. F., & Pedreira, M. E. (2020). Psychological distress associated with COVID-19 quarantine: Latent profile analysis, outcome prediction and mediation analysis. *Journal of Affective Disorders*, 277: 75–84.

Frontera, J. A., Yang, D., Lewis, A., Patel, P., Medicherla, C., Arena, V., Fang, T., Andino, A., Snyder, T., Madhavan, M., Gratch, D., Fuchs, B., Dessy, A., Canizares, M., Jauregui, R., Thomas, B., Bauman, K., Olivera, A., Bhagat, D., Sonson, M., Park, G., Stainman, R., Sunwoo, B., Talmasov, D., Tamimi, M., Zhu, Y., Rosenthal, J., Dygert, L., Ristic, M., Ishii, H., Valdes, E., Omari, M., Gurin, L., Huang, J., Czeisler, B. M., Kahn, D. E., Zhou, T., Lin, J., Lord, A. S., Melmed, K., Meropol, S., Troxel, A. B., Petkova, E., Wisniewski, T., Balcer, L., Morrison, C., Yaghi, S., & Galetta S. (2021). A prospective study of long-term outcomes among hospitalized COVID-19 patients with and without neurological complications. *Journal of Neurological Science*, 426: 117486. doi: 10.1016/j.jns.2021.117486

Gaeta, L., & Brydges, C. R. (2020). Coronavirus-related anxiety, social isolation, and loneliness in older adults in Northern California during the stay-at-home order. *Journal of Aging and Social Policy*, 33(4–5): 320–331.

García-Fernández, L., Romero-Ferreiro, V., Padilla, S., López-Roldán, P. D., Monzó-García, M., & Rodigruez-Jimenez, R. (2020). Gender differences in emotional responses to the COVID-19 outbreak in Spain. *Brain and Behavior*, 11(1): e09134. 10.1002/brb3.1934

Goldberg, L. R. (1993). The structure of phenotypic personality traits. *American Psychologist*, 48(1): 26–34.

Goldmann, E., & Galea, S. (2014). Mental health consequences of disasters. *Annual Review of Public Health*, 35: 169–183. doi: 10.1146/annurev-publhealth-032013-182435

Grant, A. M., Curtayne, L., & Burton, G. (2009). Executive coaching enhances goal attainment, resilience and workplace well-being: A randomised controlled study. *The Journal of Positive Psychology*, 4(5): 396–407.

Hamel, L., & Salganikoff, A. (2020, 6th April.) Is there a widening gender gap in coronavirus stress? KFF. Retrieved from: https://www.kff.org/policy-watch/is-there-widening-gender-gap-in-coronavirus-stress/

Hampshire, A., Trender, W., Chamberlain, S. R., Jolly, A. E., Grant, J. E., Patrick, F., Mazibuko, N., Williams, S. C., Barnby, J. M., Hellyer, P., & Mehta, M. A. (2021). Cognitive deficits in people who have recovered from COVID-19. *EClinicalMedicine*, 39: 101044. doi: 10.1016/j.eclinm.2021.101044

Han, J., & Richardson, V. E. (2010). The relationship between depression and loneliness among homebound older persons: Does spirituality moderate this relationship? *Journal of Religion and Spirituality in Social Work*, 29: 218–236. doi: 10.1080/15426432.2010.495610

Hawker, M., & Romero-Ortuno, R. (2016). Social determinants of discharge outcomes in older people admitted to a geriatric medicine ward. *Journal of Frailty & Aging*, 5(2):118–12010.14283/jfa.2016.897

Hawkley, L. C., Thisted, R. A., Masi, C. M., & Cacioppo, J. T. (2010). Loneliness predicts increased blood pressure: 5-year cross-lagged analyses in middle-aged and older adults. *Psychology and Aging*, 25(1): 132–141.

Heffner, K. L., Waring, M. E., Roberts, M. B., Eaton, C. B., & Gramling, R. (2011). Social isolation, C-reactive protein, and coronary heart disease mortality among community-dwelling adults. *Social Science and Medicine*, 72: 1482–1488. doi: 10.1016/j.socscimed.2011.03.016

Horesh, D., Kapel Lev-Ari, R., & Hasson-Ohayon, I. (2020). Risk factors for psychological distress during the COVID-19 pandemic in Israel: Loneliness, age, gender, and health status play an important role. *British Journal of Health Psychology*, 25: 925–933.

Hou, F., Bi, F., Jiao, R. et al. (2020). Gender differences of depression and anxiety among social media users during the COVID-19 outbreak in China: A cross-sectional study. *BMC Public Health*, 20: 1648. 10.1186/s12889-020-09738-7

Huang, M., Wang, H., Wang, G., Liu, Z., & Hu, S. (2020). Factors associated with mental health outcomes among health care workers exposed to coronavirus disease 2019. *JAMA Network Open*, 3(3), e203976. doi: 10.1001/jamanetworkopen.2020.3976

Hyland, R., Rochford, S., Munnelly, A., Dodd, P., Fox, R., Vallières, F., McBride, O., Shevlin, M., Bentall, Richard P., Butter, S., Karatzias, T., & Murphy, J. (2021). Predicting risk along the suicidality continuum: A longitudinal, nationally representative study of the Irish population during the COVID-19 pandemic. *Suicide and Life-Threatening Behavior*, 52(1): 83–98.

Jia, R., Ayling, K., Chalder, T., Massey, A., Broadbent, E., Coupland, C., et al. (2020). Mental health in the UK during the COVID-19 pandemic: Early observations. *Frontiers in Psychiatry*, 12: 650759. doi: 10.3389/fpsyt.2021.650759

Kestilä, L., Härmä, V., & Rissanen, V. (2020). COVID-19-epidemian vaikutukset hyvinvointiin, palvelujärjestelmään ja kansantalouteen. In The Implications of COVID-19 to Wellbeing, Service Systems and Economy; Expert Assessment, Report 14/20; Finnish Institute of Health and Welfare: Helsinki, Finland.

Leigh-Hunt, N., Bagguley, D., Rash, K., Turner, V., Turnbull, S., Valtorta, N., et al. (2017). An overview of systematic reviews on the public health consequences of social isolation and loneliness. *Public Health*, 152: 157–171.

Liang, Y., Wu, K., Zhou, Y., Huang, X., Zhou, Y., & Liu, Z. (2020). Mental health in frontline medical workers during the 2019 novel coronavirus disease epidemic in China: A comparison with the general population. *International Journal of Environmental Research and Public Health*, 17(18): 6550. doi: 10.3390/ijerph17186550

Liotta, E. M., Batra, A., Clark, J. R., Shlobin, N. A., Hoffman, S. C., Orban, Z. S., & Koranilk, I. J. (2020). Frequent neurological manifestations and encephalopathy-associated morbidity in Covid-19 patients. *Annals of Clinical and Translational Neurology*, 7(11): 2221–2230.

López-Núñez, M. I., Díaz-Morales, J. F., & Aparicio-García, M. E. (2020). Individual differences, personality, social, family and work variables on mental health during COVID-19 outbreak in Spain. *Personality and Individual Differences*, 172: 110562

Ma, Z., Zhao, J., Li, Y., Chen, D., Wang, T., Zhang, Z., Chen, Z., Yu, Q., Jiang, J., Fan, F., & Liu, X. (2020). Mental health problems and correlates among 746 217 college students during the coronavirus disease 2019 outbreak in China. *Epidemiology and Psychiatric Sciences*, 29: e181. doi: 10.1017/S2045796020000931

Mazza, C., Ricci, E., Biondi, S., Colasanti, M., Ferracuti, S., Napoli, C., & Roma, P. (2020). A nationwide survey of psychological distress among Italian people during the COVID-19 pandemic: Immediate psychological responses and associated factors. *International Journal of Environmental Research and Public Health*, 17(9): 3185.

McCrae, R. R., & Costa, P. T. (1987). Validation of the five-factor model of personality across instruments and observers. *Journal of Personality and Social Psychology*. 52 (1): 81–90.

McGinty, E. E., Presskreischer, R., Anderson, K. E., Han, H., & Barry, C. L. (2020a). Psychological distress and COVID-19-related stressors reported in a longitudinal cohort of US adults in April and July 2020. *JAMA*, 324(24): 2555–2557. doi: 10.1001/jama.2020.21231

McGinty, E. E., Presskreischer, R., Han, H., & Barry, C. L. (2020b). Psychological distress and loneliness reported by US adults in 2018 and April 2020. *JAMA*, 324: 93–94. doi: 10.1001/jama.2020.9740

McManus, S., Bebbington, P., Jenkins, R., & Brugha, T. (Eds.) (2016). *Mental health and well-being in England: Adult Psychiatric Morbidity Study 2014*. NatCen Social Research Centre and the Department of Health Services, University of Leicester for NHS Digital. Leeds, UK: NHS Digital. Retrieved from: https://assets.publishing.service.gov.uk/government/uploads/system/uploads/attachment_data/file/556596/apms-2014-full-rpt.pdf

Mental Health Foundation (2020, 9th July). Coronavirus: The divergence of mental health experiences during the pandemic. Available at: https://www.mentalhealth.org.uk/coronavirus/divergence-mental-health-experiences-during-pandemic

Mohammadpour, M., Ghorbani, V., Khoramnia, S., Ahmadi, S. M., Ghvami, M., &, Maleki, M. (2020). Anxiety, self-compassion, gender differences and COVID-19: Predicting self-care behaviors and fear of COVID-19 based on anxiety and self-compassion with an emphasis on gender differences. *Iran Journal of Psychiatry*, 15(3): 213–219. doi:10.18502/ijps.v15i3.3813

Nikcevic, A. V., Marino, C., Kolubinski, D. C., Leach, D., & Spada, M. M. (2020). Modelling the contribution of the Big Five personality traits, health anxiety, and COVID-19 psychological distress to generalised anxiety and depressive symptoms during the COVID-19 pandemic. *Journal of Affective Disorders*, 279: 578–584.

Office for National Statistics (2020, 19th June). Coronavirus and the social impacts on Great Britain. Retrieved from: https://www.ons.gov.uk/releases/coronavirusandthesocialimpactsongreatbritain19june2020

Office for National Statistics (2021, 10th March). Coroavirus (COVID-19) and the different effects on men and women in the UK, March 2030 to April 2021. Retrieved from: https://www.ons.gov.uk/peoplepopulationandcommunity/healthandsocialcare/conditionsanddiseases/articles/coronaviruscovid19andthedifferenteffectsonmenandwomenintheukmarch2020tofebruary2021/2021-03-10

Ostacoli, L., Cosma, S., Bevilacqua, F., Berchialla, P., Bovetti, M., Carosso, A. R., Malandrone, F., Carletto, S., & Benedetto, C. (2020). Psychosocial factors associated with postpartum psychological distress during the Covid-19 pandemic: A cross-sectional study. *BMC Pregnancy Childbirth*, 20(1): 703. doi: 10.1186/s12884-020-03399-5

O'Connor, R. C., Wetherall, K., Cleare, S., McClelland, H., Melson, A. J., Niedzwiedz, C. L., O'Carroll, R. E., O'Connor, D. B., Platt, S., Scowcroft, E., Watson, B., Zortea, T., Ferguson, E., & Robb, K. A. (2020). Mental health and well-being during the COVID-19 pandemic: longitudinal analyses of adults in the UK COVID-19 Mental Health & Wellbeing study. *The British Journal of Psychiatry*, 218(6): 326–33310.1192/bjp.2020.212

Pakenham, K. I., Landi, G., Boccolini, G., Furlani, A., Grandi, S., & Tossani, E. (2020). The moderating roles of psychological flexibility and inflexibility on the mental health impacts of COVID-19 pandemic and lockdown in Italy. *Journal of Contextual Behavioural Science*, 17: 109–118.

Pierce, M., Hope, H., Ford, T., Hatch, S., Hotopf, M., John. A., Kontopantelis, E., Webb, R., Wessely, S., McManus, S., & Abel, K. (2020). Mental health before and during the COVID-19 pandemic: A longitudinal probability sample survey of the UK population. *Lancet Psychiatry*, (10): 883–892. doi: 10.1016/S2215-0366(20)30308-4

Pierce, M., McManus, S., Jessop, C., John, A., Hotopf, M., Ford, T., Hatch, S., Wessely, S., & Abel, K. M. (2020). Says who? The significance of sampling in mental health surveys during COVID-19. *Lancet Psychiatry*, 7(7): 567–568. doi: 10.1016/S2215-0366(20)30237-6

Planchuelo-Gómez, Á., Odriozola-González, P., Irurtia, M. J., & De Luis-García, R. (2020). Longitudinal evaluation of the psychological impact of the COVID-19 crisis in Spain. *Journal of Affective Disorders*, 277: 842–849.

Porter, C., Favara, M., Hittmeyer, A., Scott, D., Sanchez Jimenez, A., Ellanki, R., Woldehanna, T., Duc, L. T., Crasks, M. G., & Stein, A. (2020). Impact of the COVID-19 pandemic on anxiety and depression symptoms of young people in the global south: Evidence from a four-country cohort study. *BMJ Open*, https://bmjopen.bmj.com/content/11/4/e049653

Pradhan, M., Chettri, A., & Maheshwari, S. (2020). Fear of death in the shadow of COVID-19: The mediating role of perceived stress in the relationship between neuroticism and death anxiety. *Death Studies*, 16, 1–5.

Preti, E., Di Mattei, V., Perego, G., Ferrari, F., Mazzetti, M., Taranto, P., Di Pierro, R., Madeddu, F., & Calati, R. (2020). The psychological impact of epidemic and pandemic outbreaks on healthcare workers: Rapid review of the evidence. *Current Psychiatry Reports*, 22(8): 43. doi: 10.1007/s11920-020-01166-z

Prowse, R., Sherratt, F., Abizaid, A., Gabrys, R. L., Hellemans, K. G. L., Patterson, Z. R., & McQuaid, R. T. (2021). Coping with the COVID-19 pandemic: Examining gender differences in stress and mental health among university students. *Frontiers in Psychiatry*. 10.3389/fpsyt.2021.650759

Ran, L., Wang, W., Ai, M., Kong, Y., Chen, J., & Kuang, L. (2020). Psychological resilience, depression, anxiety, and somatization symptoms in response to COVID-19: A study of the general population in China at the peak of its epidemic. *Social Science and Medicine*, 262: 113261

Renner, R. (2020, 15th April). The pandemic is giving people vivid, unusual dreams. Here's why. National Geographic. Retrieved from: https://www.nationalgeographic.co.uk/science-and-technology/2020/04/pandemic-giving-people-vivid-unusual-dreams-heres-why

Rettie, H., & Daniels, J. (2020). Coping and tolerance of uncertainty: Predictors and mediators of mental health during the COVID-19 pandemic. *American Psychologist*, 3rd August. Doi: 10.1037/amp0000710

Ritchie, K., Chan, D., & Watermeyer, T. (2020). The cognitive consequences of the COVID-19 epidemic: Collateral damage? *Brain Communication*, 2(2): fcaa069. doi:10.1093/braincomms/fcaa069

Rogers, J. P., Chesney, E., Oliver, D., Poliak, T. A., McGuire, P., Fusar-Poli, P., Zandi, M. S., Lewis, G., & David, A. S. (2020). Psychiatric and neuropsychiatric presentations associated with severe coronavirus infections: A systematic review and meta-analysis with comparison to the COVID-19 pandemic. *Lancet Psychiatry*, 7(7): 611–727.

Roma, P., Monaro, M., Colasanti, M., Ricci, E., Biondi, S., Di Domenico, A., Verrocchio, M. C., Napoli, C., Ferracuti, S., & Mazza, C. A. (2020). 2-Month follow-up study of psychological distress among Italian People during the COVID-19 Lockdown. *International Journal of Environmental Research and Public Health*, 17(21): 8180. doi: 10.3390/ijerph17218180

Ruiz-Frutos, C., Ortega-Moreno, M., Allande-Cussó, R., Ayuso-Murillo, D., Domínguez-Salas, S., & Gómez-Salgado, J. (2021). Sense of coherence, engagement, and work environment as precursors of psychological distress among non-health workers during the COVID-19 pandemic in Spain. *Safety Science*, 133: 105033. 10.1016/j.ssci.2020.105033

Samitarians (2019, December). Suicide statistics report: Latest statistics for the UK and Republic of Ireland. Retrieved from: https://media.samaritans.org/documents/SamaritansSuicideStatsReport_2019_Full_report.pdf

Savolainen, I., Oksa, R., Savela, N., Celuch, M., & Oksanen, A. (2021). COVID-19 anxiety – A longitudinal survey study of psychological and situational risks among Finnish workers. *International Journal of Environmental Research and Public Health*, 18: 794. DOI: 10.3390/ijerph18020794

Shankar, A., McMunn, A., Banks, J., & Steptoe, A. (2011). Loneliness, social isolation, and behavioral and biological health indicators in older adults. *Health Psychology*, 30: 377–385. doi: 10.1037/a0022826

Shevlin, M., Butter, S., McBride, O., Murphy, J., Gibson-Miller, J., Hartman, T. K., Levita, L., Mason, L., Martinez, A. P., McKay, R., Stocks, T. V. A., Bennett, K., Hyland, P., & Bentall, R. (2021). Refuting the myth of a 'tsunami' of mental ill-health in populations affected by COVID-19: Evidence that response to the pandemic is heterogeneous, not homogeneous. *Psychological Medicine*. Advanced online publication. doi:10.1017/S0033291721001665

Shevlin, M., McBride, O., Murphy, J., Miller, J. G., Hartman, T. K., Levita, L., Mason, L., Martinez, A. P., McKay, R., Stocks, T. V. A., Bennett, K. M., Hyland, P., Karatzias, T., & Bentall, R. P. (2020, 19 October). Anxiety, depression, traumatic stress and COVID-19-related anxiety in the UK general population during the COVID-19 pandemic. *British Journal of Psychology Open*, 6(6): e125. doi: 10.1192/bjo.2020.109

Shi, L., Lu, Z. A., Que, J. Y., Huang, X. L., Liu, L., Ran, M. S., Gong, Y. M., Yuan, K., Yan, W., Sun, Y. K., Shi, J., Bao, Y. P., & Lu, L. (2020). Prevalence of and risk factors associated with mental health symptoms among the general population in China during the coronavirus disease 2019 Pandemic. *JAMA Network Open*, 3(7): e2014053. doi: 10.1001/jamanetworkopen.2020.14053

Somma, A., Gialdi, G., Krueger, R. F., Markon, K. E., Frau, C., Lovallo, S., & Fossati, A. (2020). Dysfunctional personality features, nonscientifically supported causal beliefs, and emotional problems during the first month of the COVID-19 pandemic in Italy. *Personality and Individual Differences*, 165: 110139.

Song, S., Yang, X., Yang, H., Zhou, P., Ma, H., Teng, C., Chen, H., Ou, H., Li, J., Mathews, C. A., Nutley, S., Liu, N., Zhang, X., & Zhang, N. (2021). Psychological resilience as a protective factor for depression and anxiety among the public during the outbreak of COVID-19. *Frontiers in Psychology*, 11: 618509. DOI: 10.3389.fpsyg.2020.618509

Talbot, J., Charron, V., & Konkle, A. T. M. (2020). Feeling the void: Lack of support for isolation and sleep difficulties in pregnant women during the COVID-19 pandemic revealed by Twitter data analysis. *International Journal of Environmental Research and Public Health*, 18(2): 393. 10.3390/ijerph18020393

Thomson, A. (2020, 21st October). Second wave is bringing a mental health crisis. *The Times*, p. 25.

Trougakos, J. P., Chawla, N., & McCarthy, J. M. (2020). Working in a pandemic: Exploring the impact of COVID-19 health anxiety on work, family, and health outcomes. *Journal of Applied Psychology*, 105: 1234–1245.

Van Rheenen, T. E., Meyer, D., Neill, E., Phillipou, A., Tan, E. J., Toh, W. L., & Rossell, S. L. (2020). Mental health status of individuals with a mood-disorder during the COVID-19 pandemic in Australia: Initial results from the COLLATE project. *Journal of Affective Disorders*, 1(275): 69–77. doi: 10.1016/j.jad.2020.06.037

Waizenegger, L., McKenna, B., Cai, W., & Bendz, T. (2020). An affordance perspective of team collaboration and enforced working from home during COVID-19. *European Journal of Information Systems*, 29: 429–442.

Wang, H. X., Mittleman, M. A., & Orth-Gomer, K. (2005). Influence of social support on progression of coronary artery disease in women. *Social Science and Medicine*, 60: 599–607.

Wang, C., Pan, R., Wan, X., Tan, Y., Xu, L., Ho, C. S., & Ho, R. C. (2020). Immediate psychological responses and associated factors during the initial stage of the 2019 coronavirus disease (COVID-19) epidemic among the general population in China. *International Journal of Environmental Research and Public Health*, 17(5): 1729. doi: 10.3390/ijerph17051729

Wang, C., Pan, R., Wan, X., Tan, Y., Xu, L., McIntyre, R. S., Choo, F. N., Tran, B., Ho, R., Sharma, V. K., et al. (2020). A longitudinal study on the mental health of general population during the COVID-19 epidemic in China. *Brain Behaviour and Immunity*, 87: 40–48.

Wathelet M., Duhem S., Vaiva G., et al. (2020). Factors associated with mental health disorders among University Students in France confined during the COVID-19 pandemic. *JAMA Network Open*, 3(10): e2025591. Published 2020 Oct 1. doi:10.1001/jamanetworkopen.2020.25591

White, T. (2020, 4th December). COVID-19's potential impact on neurological function and mental health. *verywellmind*. Retrieved from: https://www.verywellmind.com/covid-19-impact-on-neurological-and-mental-health-5088603

Wielgus, B., Urban, W., Patriak, A., & Cichocki, Ł. (2020). Examining the associations between psychological flexibility, mindfulness, psychosomatic functioning, and anxiety during the COVID-19 pandemic: A path analysis. *International Journal of Environmental Research and Public Health*, 17: 8764.

Winkler P., Formanek T., Mlada K., Kagstrom A., Mohrova Z., Mohr P., & Csemy L. (2020 Sep 29). Increase in prevalence of current mental disorders in the context of COVID-19: Analysis of repeated nationwide cross-sectional surveys. *Epidemiology and Psychiatric Science*, 29:e173. doi: 10.1017/S2045796020000888

Xu, J., Ou, J., Luo, S., Wang, Z., Chang, E., Novak, C., Shen, J., Zheng, S., & Wang, Y. (2020). Perceived social support protects lonely people against COVID-19 anxiety: A three-wave longitudinal study in China. *Frontiers of Psychology*. Retrieved from: 10.3389/fpsyg.2020.566965

Xue, B., & McMunn, A. (2020). Gender differences in the impact of the Covid-19 lockdown on unpaid care work and psychological distress in the UK. *PLoS One*, 6(3):e0247959. doi: 10.1371/journal.pone.0247959

Yamamoto, T., Uchiumi, Suzuki, N., Yoshimoto, J., & Murillo-Rodriguez, E. (2020). The psychological impact of 'Mild Lockdown' in Japan during the COVID-10 pandemic: A nationwide survey under a declared state of emergency. *International Journal of Environmental Research and Public Health*, 17(24): 9382. doi: 10.3390/ijerph17249382

YouGov (2020a, 9th October). What impact would you say that the coronavirus pandemic has had, if at all, on your mental health. Available at: https://yougov.co.uk/topics/health/survey-results/daily/2020/10/09/26286/2

YouGov (2020b, 9th October). How often, if at all, have you felt lonely in the last two months? Available at: https://yougov.co.uk/topics/health/survey-results/daily/2020/10/09/26286/3

Zhang, Y., & Ma, Z. F. (2020). Impact of the COVID-19 pandemic on mental health and quality of life among local residents in Liaoning Province, China: A cross-sectional study. *International Journal of Environmental Research and Public Health*, 17(7): 2381. doi: 10.3390/ijerph17072381

Chapter 5

COVID-19, Mental Health and the Young

By April 2020, schools had been suspended nationwide in 188 countries as the pandemic spread at an accelerating rate. This meant that the learning of 1.5 billion young people had been disrupted (UNESCO, 2020). Experts warned of the vulnerability of adolescents to adverse mental health reactions in a crisis situation such as the pandemic (Busby, 2020). Prior research with this age group indicated that the uncertainty created by the pandemic, dramatic and fundamental changes to their everyday routines and involuntary confinement to home would all represent stressors and were likely in many cases eventually to motivate push-back against restrictions (Viner et al., 2021).

Evidence collected from around the world, from high-, middle- and low-income countries showed that school closures could cause a variety of health-related and safety-related issues for children. In some regions, schools were sources of nutrition and when closed resulted in poorer diets for the children affected. Elsewhere, children's personal safety was put at risk by spending more time out of school. In other places, there was a depletion in children's life satisfaction and an increase in mental health issues including anxiety and depression (Rajmil et al., 2021).

One major review of 80 studies mainly from Australia, China, Europe and the United States show that loneliness was linked to mental health and found small to moderate associations between social isolation and loneliness and moderate associations between social isolation/loneliness and general anxiety (Loades et al., 2020).

Increased dependence on media technologies and online communications systems – already so central to their lives – might also enhance the likelihood of exposure to potentially upsetting content. There was an expectation therefore that this age group might suffer mentally, even though not a high-risk group in terms of physical infection and associated serious illness (Guessoum et al., 2020).

DOI: 10.4324/9781003274377-5

Global Public Opinion about Mental Health Impact of Pandemic on Children

Plenty of evidence emerged that parents believed the pandemic and ac-companying school closures had had a significant impact on the mental health and general well-being of children and that these effects might be felt for some time after the pandemic was over. Although such data does not represent evidence of the actual impacts of the pandemic on children, it is important in presenting a general picture of the climate of concern that had materialised around the world.

In a poll of over 20,000 people in 29 countries of public perceptions of the impact of the pandemic on children by Ipsos-MORI in May and early June 2021, nearly four in ten people (37%) thought that the pandemic would have lasting effects on the mental health and well-being of children and young people. This concern was least likely to be voiced in South Korea (19%), but more widely in the United Kingdom (45%), Sweden (51%) and Canada (50%) (Beaver et al., 2021, 15th July).

At the same time, more than six in ten people (62%), on average, regarded school closures as an acceptable price to pay to protect children and others from COVID-19, though this opinion varied widely across countries. It was most widely endorsed in Mexico (81%), Peru (81%), Colombia (80%) and Chile (79%) and least widely held in South Korea (38%), Japan (41%) and Italy (42%). In Britain, it was endorsed by two-thirds of respondents (68%), but by notably fewer than this in the United States (58%).

Around four in ten people across the globe felt that children and young people would probably experience difficulties concentrating again once they returned to school. Around one in three (32%), on average, foresaw pro-blems getting students to reintegrate with each other and with their teachers upon returning to schools and the same proportion (32%) also predicted difficulties instilling good behaviour and discipline again. These were, of course, minority opinions and many other parents were less concerned about any side-effects of this sort (Beaver et al., 2021).

Direct Evidence of Mental Health Effects

Some children and young people may have had a history of mental health problems before the pandemic. For these, it was important to consider whether they were especially at risk from the suspension of the usual sources of support during the lockdown. A survey of over 2,000 young people in the United Kingdom aged up to 25 with a history of mental health problems found that most (83%) felt the pandemic had made their condition worse. Equally concerning, one in four (26%) claimed they had been unable to obtain any support as usual services had been cancelled and no remote access substitutes had been made readily available.

The impact of school closures can be far-reaching. When children go to school, teachers take over child-minding responsibilities for a large part of the day. Remove that service and parents must make alternative arrangements that might not only be inconvenient but also costly. Schools also offer many children and teenagers structure and routine in their lives. Once this is taken away, many may experience serious difficulties knowing how to cope. In a crisis situation in which they are also required to socially isolate, they might withdraw into their bedrooms and without supportive social contact, anxiety and depression symptoms can be seeded, especially among those with a predisposition to react in this way (Lee, 2020).

For adolescents that have reached a stage in their education where they are starting to plan for what comes next, social distancing protocols can prove to be particularly worrying when the future becomes unclear. Many universities around the world suspended entrance procedures leaving final-year students in schools adrift, not knowing when they might continue their education and increasingly concerned about their eventual career prospects.

In Switzerland, Shanahan, Steinhoff, Bechtiger, Murray and others (2020) found clear signs of increased stress and feelings of anger among young adult respondents during the pandemic compared with pre-pandemic levels. Those who had already reported emotional distress before the pandemic displayed even greater distress symptoms during it. Other life stressors included uncertainty about future employment, reduced income during the pandemic, social deprivation and fears about the new virus. Disruption to education and loss of employment emerged as powerful predictors of pandemic-related stress across the sample. These were generally more powerful predictors of emotional distress during the pandemic than were health-related fears.

Psychologists and psychiatrists noted both that the pandemic would be a major stressor for young people and an opportunity to study the impact of non-pharmaceutical interventions focused on the mental health of children and adolescents. For all the attention being given to modelling behaviour to combat the spread of the disease, it is important to recognise that these intervention "solutions" could cause severe health problems of their own (Bruining et al., 2020; Courtney et al., 2020).

Lockdown and the Psychological Health of Young People

Children and young adults still in full-time education were among the groups significantly affected by lockdowns during the COVID-19 pandemic. Research from different parts of the world found that students reported having been seriously impacted by the pandemic. Their universities frequently closed many of their usual services to students. Much or indeed all face-to-face teaching halted for months on end and online tuition was offered instead. Many universities struggled to get to grips with this alternative form of teaching and even when it was done well, it failed to compensate fully for normal face-to-face teaching formats. Moreover, the closure of many facilities on campuses meant that students missed the important social dimension of the university experience.

Pre-COVID-pandemic research had shown that social isolation in childhood can contribute towards the development of mental health issues in young people. Loneliness was known to trigger anxiety symptoms and even more research had shown that it was linked to childhood depression (Loades et al., 2020). Losing contact with friends and peer groups is a particularly terrible blow for adolescents who turn to these sources for a definition of their own social identity (Leary, 1990). Young people can feel excluded when their social contacts are cut off (Beck & Clark, 1988). Under social isolation conditions, there is a generic threat to social relationships and to the social status they might confer on the individual (Wiseman, 2008).

Research in Canada showed that teenagers reported feelings of loneliness and depression after their schools had been closed in response to the pandemic. These youngsters were very concerned about COVID-19, but their concerns extended beyond personal risks of infection. They were worried about getting behind with their school work and about not being able to see their friends, other than via technology. Evidence emerged that connecting with friends via social media sites and spending more time physically with their immediate family did help to stave off loneliness and also allowed some to develop close relationships even more than they would under normal living conditions. These relationships did provide valuable social support, but this was not a complete substitute for face-to-face contact and being able to leave home more freely (Ellis et al., 2020).

Further empirical evidence emerged that COVID-19 and the actions taken by the government to combat it had taken their toll on young people. In some cases, the mental impact of the pandemic derived from becoming infected by COVID-19 and on other occasions, it was triggered by the many disruptions to the lives of children and adolescents caused by the pandemic. Common effects were increased anxiety, depression and post-traumatic stress (Petrosillo et al., 2020; World Health Organization, 2020).

Similar findings had been found to occur among children during earlier pandemics (Cheng et al., 2004; Chua et al., 2004; Cheng & Wong, 2005). These effects can sometimes last for a long time (Mak et al., 2009). Hence, the risks to children's general health and well-being caused by pandemics and the use of extensive non-pharmaceutical measures to control them were not unknown before the COVID-19 pandemic. Yet, these experiences and lessons learned from them did not extend around the world. That was probably the main reason why many countries that had remained only lightly touched by earlier, recent pandemics were not prepared when a major pandemic struck them directly.

While young people, in some parts of the world, had previously experienced psychologically damaging side-effects of pandemics, none of those had achieved the scale of the COVID-19 pandemic. Understandably therefore researchers around the world have shown a lot of concern about the eventual impact it will have in the longer term on young people's lives and especially their mental health (Ghosh et al., 2020; Viner et al., 2020; Wang et al., 2020).

In devising urgent strategies to combat the pandemic, many national governments deployed a wide range of interventions and many of these, most notably, instructions to stay at home, not to see friends, and the closure of schools, had a significant impact on children. Parents and carers might often do what they can to protect their children from the stress that having their lives curtailed in this way could trigger. Yet, in taking this stress upon themselves, parents' anxieties might become apparent to their children who then worry anyway (Mackler et al., 2015; Sanner & Neece, 2018; Ellis et al., 2020; Thomas, 2020).

The loss of their usual routine and restrictions that permit only remote, electronic communications with their friends could trigger feelings of loneliness in some children and cause frustration in others. If they persist these feelings could evolve into more serious mental health conditions. Research evidence emerged that between a fifth and third of children in studies from around the world reported experiencing increased anxiety during the pandemic. Other evidence emerged of children experiencing depression symptoms. In some studies, the prevalence of depression reached exceeded two-fifths of the youngsters questioned (Loades et al., 2020; Liu et al., 2020; Secer & Ulas, 2020; Zhou et al., 2020).

The interventions themselves might also trigger mental health symptoms. So, as well as worrying about the risks of infection, having their usual behaviour patterns curtailed for an uncertain length of time can leave some, if not many children feeling cast adrift of their normal life structures and social support systems. During the COVID pandemic, one group of researchers found that adolescents would socially distance themselves from others to protect against infection but that this specific behaviour was, in turn, related to the onset of anxiety symptoms (Oosterhoff et al., 2020). Despite understanding the importance of social distancing and other restrictions on their normal movements, compliance with these new behavioural rules could cause children and teenagers considerable distress (Burhamah et al., 2020; Nearchou et al., 2020; Trzebinski et al., 2020).

Young People, Families and COVID-19

The coronavirus pandemic presented a number of challenges to families, social networks, schools and local communities. The social dynamics with which children can engage with each of these groups underpins their resilience in life. This means that children's awareness of how to behave and how to overcome specific problems they might face in later life derive from social learning with these groups. The disruption of regular social structures during pandemic lockdowns meant that children's lives lacked the stability and the certainty that was normal to them (BPS, 2020, 23rd June).

Schools in particular cultivated a sense of belonging in children, independent of what they had acquired from their families. For some children, schools might have offered greater stability than their home life. Schools offer children structure and routine and when they were closed not only was regular ordinary, everyday life suspended, it was for many totally disrupted. It was not just a matter of their education being held back, although that was serious enough. It was also the fact that the structure that schools provided for a significant portion of their waking hours each weekday was no longer available and found no effective substitute anywhere else.

Being taken out of school could therefore be the source of considerable anxiety. This new anxiousness could be compounded with the pressure some children already experience at school where they had to work hard to stay on top of their schoolwork and also in some cases had to deal with less than friendly relationships with other students. Being at home, with their education disrupted caused children anxiety. Over time, however, they might have learned to cope with this new scenario to a degree that anxiety was triggered again when they returned to school. For some, their concerns might also have been underpinned by uncertainty over how safe it was to go back to school. For children with special educational needs, the withdrawal of special, professional support could be especially troubling both for the students and their families (Lee, 2020). The subject of school closures is examined in more detail later in this chapter.

School Closures and Children's Mental Health

Among the organisations affected by these new rules were universities and schools. Many or all were required to close or to observe strict physical distancing and hygiene protocols if they remained opened. There is nothing new in adopting this kind of intervention when pandemics strike (Public Health England, 2014; New Zealand Ministry of Health, 2017). There were understandable concerns about the impact of such closures on the educational development of young people. As already noted, there were concerns about the deployment of school closures as an intervention (Lee, 2020). Pupils were not the only ones to feel anxious. Teachers and other support staff also had to contend with fears that they might be exposed to the novel coronavirus back at work (Muller & Goldenberg, 2020). Many teachers reported going onto medication and seeking professional help during the pandemic because of uncertainties and pressures linked to their job during the pandemic

(Busby, 2021, 3rd April). Hence, there was a need for support strategies and systems to assist all relevant stakeholders – staff and pupils at school.

Previous research had provided mixed evidence concerning its effectiveness as a non-pharmaceutical intervention during a runaway pandemic, even it was efficacious in reducing opportunities for the spread of an infectious virus, it could also cause considerable collateral damage to the lives of children, parents and teachers and also to the future educational fitness of an entire nation (Markel et al., 2007; Cowling et al., 2008; Cauchemez et al., 2009; Jackson et al., 2014a, 2014b; Rashid et al., 2015).

Alternative forms of tuition were proposed which included remote virtual learning practices and in the case of children, the involvement of parents in "home schooling". Many educational establishments, however, were caught napping by this sudden turn of events.

Adolescents were found to make the most of a bad situation but sometimes struggled psychologically to cope with the pressures experienced during the pandemic. For many, being separated from their friends, their schools and from their everyday lives was less than ideal. Some compensated with more substance abuse, but this was not the norm. There were tensions at home, especially with parents. At the same time, those who might have been targets for bullying or unflattering treatment gained some relief as this behaviour largely disappeared while pandemic-related restrictions were in place. The lack of control over their everyday lives and the general uncertainties created by the pandemic did put a strain on the mental health of many, and especially girls (Kapetanovic et al., 2021). Adolescence is normally a time when individuals experience heightened psychological issues. The uncertainties of the pandemic merely added to the stresses usually associated with this important period of psychological development.

After the coronavirus disease started to take hold in China, the government closed schools across the country and discouraged public activities. At one point it was estimated that 220 million Chinese children were confined to their homes. These children were served by an emergency home schooling plan. Schools created and delivered online courses and used television broadcasts and the internet to deliver them. The aim was to provide an effective substitute for normal schooling that would minimise any damage to children's education caused by the lockdown. It was also designed to assure and give support to parents who were concerned for their children.

Despite all these best efforts, there was concern that the prolonged school closures would have an adverse psychological impact on children and that their mental health might suffer. There was also evidence that children were less physically active when they did not go to school, resulting in poorer physical fitness, spending more time watching screens (not just for educational reasons), sleeping more poorly and having poorer diets which also presented a risk of weight gain (Wang et al., 2020).

Being confined to home for a long time without direct social contact, persistent fear of infection, lack of personal space at home and financial problems caused by parents losing employment together presented a cocktail of stressors that impact on the youngest family members. Some children experienced considerable distress in these conditions and this stayed with them for a long time, even when quarantining restrictions were lifted.

Governments were advised to recognise these consequences as serious. Further interventions were believed to be necessary to mitigate against them and schools and parents have parts to play in this process. Government and their education advisors could issue guidelines regarding children's educational requirements, but these need to be workable both for schools and parents or carers. Remote delivery of courses had to meet required educational standards and be engaging for students. The extent to which teachers and parents/carers needed to establish a partnership in course delivery also needed to be spelled out. At the same time, recognition had to be given to realities on the ground. For some parents, their own work commitments might have been so pressing that they could spare little time to become substitute teachers. Further, conditions at home might not have provided a comfortable education setting.

The advice could be given about how to create an effective learning environment and support materials could be produced by schools for parents and their children to use. The advice sometimes went beyond educational outcomes to include tips for making sure children get properly rested, for pacing workloads, for taking physical exercise and relating to diet. The resources of each family home ultimately determined' the degree to which each household could deliver these principles.

Further research in China, which was ahead of the rest of the world in the progress of the pandemic presented further evidence from early in this crisis to showed that the disruption it caused had pronounced psychological effects on young people. Restrictions on the movements of students in cities such as Huangshi and Wuhan in China lasted for two to three months between January and April 2020. Over this time, they were required to stay at home. They could not go to school and they could not physically socialise with their friends. One study of a large sample of children from these cities found that over one in five (23%) reported feeling depressed and nearly one in five (19%) also said they felt anxious. These figures were higher than those reported from other parts of China where behavioural restrictions had not been so severe or long-lasting. The findings were taken to be indicative of a potential mental health coronavirus pandemic (Xie et al., 2020).

Elsewhere research showed that even before the pandemic signs of growing levels of stress and anger had been detected among adolescents and those who had struggled psychologically the most with this stage of their development also experienced the greater coping difficulties once the pandemic hit. The more adolescents had experienced pre-pandemic bullying, stressful life events and feelings of social exclusion, the more they also suffered psychologically during the pandemic. Their anxieties were fuelled by a combination of uncertainty about the future, loss of control, being socially isolated from others and concern for their own health and that of their loved ones (Shanahan et al., 2020).

Thus, while young people were actually the least at risk from serious illness with COVID-19, the impact of nations' reactions to the pandemic in the form of widespread restrictions on everyday behaviour, was felt mentally to a significant degree. Some young people openly manifested their frustration by openly flouting the behavioural restrictions, but what was perhaps more potentially damaging in the longer term was the tendency among many to internalise these frustrations, allowing them to generate chronic anxiety (Reger et al., 2020).

University Closures and Students' Mental Health

In universities, the suspension of campus teaching meant that students were unable to enjoy the usual university experience and yet most were still expected to pay the same tuition fees (Stayner, 2020; Vinall, 2020). Senior university figures defended their position by claiming that students would still receive high-quality training and that their facilities needed to be maintained at considerable expense.

For students, there were serious concerns that their degrees would be devalued under this new teaching regime and that this would impact upon their future career prospects was a source of anxiety. With many then being locked away in university accommodation centres, prohibited from much socialising with other students, and in some locations forbidden to leave the premises at all, the psychological damage to their well-being was, for some, profound and potentially long-lasting. Some students felt pandemic pressure more than others. Those on courses in the physical and medical sciences, in which clinical and laboratory training could not readily be substituted by online alternatives, there was little compensation available in terms of the protection of essential learning experiences (Bentata, 2020).

The pandemic had created an extremely challenging and difficult situation for universities, and as will become clear, research emerged to show that students did experience psychological problems as a result. What is even more troubling is that university students were already known to represent an "at risk" sub-group of the wider population (Prince, 2015; Shackle, 2019). This risk was not an outcome of the physical effects of COVID-19, because they were among the least at-risk groups for infection and more especially for serious illness requiring hospital treatment. Their risk classification stemmed from how they could be expected to react mentally to the implementation of interventions designed to control the spread of the virus. A population is already known to display high levels of psychological problems could be expected to be vulnerable to the stress caused by unprecedented changes to normal university life (Stallman, 2010; Larcombe et al., 2014; Browne et al., 2017).

Studies from around the world confirmed that students experienced high anxiety specifically in response to the impact of the pandemic. Research with medical and doctoral students in Australia found that they reported feeling stressed over the disruption to their studies which could have a longer-term impact on their career prospects and personal finances (Johnson et al., 2020; Lyons et al., 2020). Research in China found that one in four (25%) students in a medical college, whose studies had been disrupted by the pandemic, felt more anxious over their coursework and being able to finish their course on time, as well as about the impact of their daily lives (Cao et al., 2020). There were reports also of international students being discriminated against or targeted as sources of infection by local populations (Zhai & Du, 2020).

Research carried out with university students in Australia, covering both domestic and international students, found that most (87%) said that their studies had been impacted by COVID-19. Only around a third (35%) claimed they were experiencing a sufficient level of well-being. Almost as many (32%) reported poor well-being. Undergraduates seemed to suffer more than did postgraduates. At all levels of study, however, there were prevalent high anxiety levels being experienced. Those who felt most strongly that the learning experience had been compromised and that their university's pandemic responses had had a huge impact on their study felt the worst. Female students seemed to feel the strain more than males (Dodd et al., 2021).

Research with Wuhan students towards the end of April 2020 found evidence of post-traumatic stress disorder. One in six (16%) reported relevant symptoms. These seemed to be aggravated by enhanced risk perceptions triggered by being away from family, worry about loss of loved ones (or actual deaths in the family) and disruption of courses (Li et al., 2021).

Lessons Learned

For children, normal amounted to going to school, being with friends, seeing members of the family that do not live with you, playing or watching sports and many other things. The pandemic meant that none of these activities was available for an indefinite period. Interviews and other conversations with children revealed that coronavirus was not always taken that seriously initially, but was seen as a bit silly. Some missed their normal routines early in the pandemic, but the novelty of living life in a different way compensated in part. Some children, often those who had fewer friends and were socially more withdrawn anyway, were able to cope better with being on their own. They would knuckle down and do their schoolwork as best they could. For others, however, lockdown presented real problems, especially after their lives had been disrupted for a few weeks. As with adults, the enforced suspension of normal life, made children reflect on what they missed and also on what they had perhaps taken for granted (Empson, 2020, 18th May).

The vast majority of children did not exhibit severe symptoms with COVID-19 once infected. Adolescents were somewhat more likely than pre-teenagers to show symptoms and were at greater risk of serious illness, but the latter risk was still small. Children and young people could still catch the virus, often with knowing they had done so and spread it to others. It was their role in a wider transmission that underpinned the use of school closures to tackle the pandemic as infection levels climbed rapidly.

As evidence reviewed in this chapter has shown, there were costs to this intervention. There was a direct impact on children's education. Schools tried to adapt to the new circumstances through the provision of remote tuition and by recruiting parents and carers into "partnerships" in which the latter would take over some of the day-to-day school workload management re-sponsibilities. This could create immense pressures within family households not least when parents themselves were struggling to adjust to working from home or to the loss of their job. Not all households had the space to create comfortable educational and working settings. For children that had reached stages in their education where important examinations were coming up, there was the additional pressure of concern about whether they could pre-pare fully without regular face-to-face contact with their teachers. This state of affairs triggered a rise of anxiety symptoms across young people who were worried they would fail their exams and then confronted with the further uncertainty of what this might mean for their futures.

The requirement to stay home also removed children from their friend-ship groups. Modern communication technologies meant that there were plenty of virtual substitutes through which they could keep in touch. Even in the digital era, however, children still benefit socially and psychologically from traditional forms of direct and physical, social interaction. Starved of this social contact and forced to cope with a new way of living in which the normal structures of the day were suspended created uncertainty and dis-ruption in children's lives that was found to have knock-on mental health effects including emotional and behavioural difficulties (Blanden et al., 2021). Such responses to the pandemic and to lockdowns were not culture specific. Research evidence quickly emerged from around the world that this was a global phenomenon. The pandemic and associated interventions on children's lives caused immediate mental health deterioration for many. This was a "known". What was not known was how long-lasting these effects might be. Potentially, the lasting impact could be considerable.

References

Aragona, M., Barbato, A., Cavani, A., Costanzo, G., & Mirisola, C. (2020). Negative impacts of COVID-19 lockdown on mental health service access and follow-up adherence for immigrants and individuals in socio-economic difficulties. *Public Health*, 186: 52–56.

Baik, C., Larcombe, W., & Brooker, A. (2019). How universities can enhance student mental wellbeing: The student perspective. *Higher Education Research and Development*, 38: 674–687.

Beaver, K., Grant-Vest, S., & Wragg, R. (2021, 15th July). New global poll finds 45% of Britons predict worse mental health and wellbeing will be one of the longest lasting outcomes of the pandemic for children. Ipsos MORI. Retrieved from: https://www.ipsos.com/ipsos-mori/en-uk/45-percent-britons-predict-worse-mental-health-wellbeing-outcomes-children

Beck, A. T. C., & Clark, D. A. (1988). Anxiety and depression: An information processing perspective. *Anxiety Research*, 88: 23–36.

Bentata, Y. (2020). The COVID-19 pandemic and international federation of medical students' association exchanges: Thousands of students deprived of their clinical and research exchanges. *Medical Education Online*, 25: 1783784.

Blanden, J., Crawford, C., Fumagalli, L., & Rabe, B. (2021, March). School closures and children's emotional and behavioural difficulties. Institute of Social & Economic Research, University of Essex. Retrieved from: https://mk0nuffieldfounpg9ee.kinstacdn.com/wp-content/uploads/2020/10/School-closures-and-childrens-emotional-and-behavioural-difficulties.pdf

BPS (2020, 23rd June). Resilience and coping: supporting transitions back to school. The British Psychological Society. Retrieved from: https://www.bps.org.uk/news-and-policy/resilience-and-coping-framework-supporting-children-going-back-school

Browne, V., Munro, J., & Cass, J. (2017). Under the Radar: The Mental Health of Australian University Students. *Journal of the Australian and New Zealand Student Services Association*, 25: 51–62.

Bruining, H., Bartels, M., Polderman, T. J., & Popma, A. (2020). COVID-19 and child and adolescent psychiatry: An unexpected blessing for part of our population? *European Child and Adolescent Psychiatry*, 30(7):1139–1140. doi: 10.1007/s00787-020-01578-5

Burhamah, W., AlKhayyat, A., Oroszlányová, M., AlKenane, A., Almansouri, A., Behbehani, M., Karimi, N., Jafar, H., & AlSuwaidan, M. (2020). The psychological burden of the COVID-19 pandemic and associated lockdown measures: Experience from 4000 participants. *Journal of Affective Disorders*, 277: 977–985.

Busby, E. (2020, 27th March). Coronavirus: Children could face more mental health problems amid lengthy school closures, experts warn. *Independent*. Retrieved from: https://www.independent.co.uk/news/education/education-news/children-mental-health-school-closure-coronavirus-childline-a9428966.html

Busby, F. (2021, 3rd April). Four in five teachers say it has affected their menta health during pandemic. *Evening Standard*. Retrieved from: https://www.standard.co.uk/news/uk/nasuwt-gavin-williamson-department-for-education-teachers-kate-green-b927693.html

Cao, W., Fang, Z., Hou, G., Han, M., Xu, X., Dong, J., & Zheng, J. (2020). The psychological impact of the COVID-19 epidemic on college students in China. *Psychiatry Research*, 287: 112934.

Casanova, M., Pagani Bagliacca, E., Silva, M., Patriarca, C., Veneroni, L., Clerici, C. A., Spreafico, F., Luksch, R., Terenziani, M., Meazza, C., et al. (2020). How young patients with cancer perceive the COVID-19 (coronavirus) epidemic in Milan, Italy: Is there room for other fears? *Pediatric Blood Cancer*, 67: e28318.

Cauchemez, S., Ferguson, N., Wachtel, C., et al. (2009). Closure of schools during an influenza pandemic. *The Lancet*, 9(8): 473–481.

Cheatley, J., Vuik, S., Devaux, M., Scarpetta, S., Pearson, M., Colombo, F., & Cecchini, M. (2020). The effectiveness of non-pharmaceutical interventions in containing epidemics: A rapid review of the literature and quantitative assessment. *medRxiv. Epub ahead of print*. DOI: 10.1101/2020.04.06.20054197

Chen, S., Jones, P. B., Underwood, B. R., Moore, A., Bullmore, E. T., Banerjee, S., Osimo, E. F., Deakin, J. B., Hatfield, C. F., Thompson, F. J., et al. (2020). The early impact of COVID-19 on mental health and community physical health services and their patients' mortality in Cambridgeshire and Peterborough, UK. *Journal of Psychiatric Research*, 131: 244–254.

Cheng, S. K. W., Tsang, J. S. K., Ku, K. H., Wong, C. W., & Ng, Y. K. (2004). Psychiatric complications in patients with severe acute respiratory syndrome (SARS) during the acute treatment phase: A series of 10 cases. *British Journal of Psychiatry*, 184: 359–360.

Cheng, S. K. W., & Wong, C. W. (2005). Psychological intervention with sufferers from severe acute respiratory syndrome (SARS): Lessons learnt from empirical findings. *Clinical Psychology and Psychotherapy*, 12: 80–86.

Chua, S. E., Cheung, V., McAlonan, G. M., Cheung, C., Wong, J. W. S., Cheung, E. P. T., Chan, M. T. Y., Wong, T. K. W., Choy, K. M., Chu, C. M., et al. (2004). Stress and psychological impact on SARS patients during the outbreak. *Canadian Journal of Psychiatry*, 49: 385–390.

Courtney, D., Watson, P., Battaglia, M., Mulsant, B. H., & Szatmari, P. (2020). COVID-19 impacts on child and youth anxiety and depression: Challenges and opportunities. *Canadian Journal of Psychiatry*, 65: 688–691.

Cowling, B. J., Lau, E. H., Lam, C. L., et al. (2008). Effects of school closures, 2008 winter influenza season, Hong Kong. *Emerging Infectious Diseases*, 14(10): 1660–1662.

de Rojas, T., Pérez-Martínez, A., Cela, E., Baragaño, M., Galán, V., Mata, C., Peretó, A., & Madero, L. (2020). COVID-19 infection in children and adolescents with cancer in Madrid. *Pediatric Blood Cancer*, 67: e28397.

Dodd, R. H., Dadaczynski, K., Okan, O., Mccaffery, K. J., & Pickles, K. (2021). Psychological wellbeing and academic experience of university students in Australia during COVID-19. *International Journal of Environmental Research and Public Health*, 18(3): 866. DOI: 10.3390/ijerph18030866

Duan, H., Yan, L., Ding, X., Gan, Y., Kohn, N., & Wu, J. (2020). Impact of the COVID-19 pandemic on mental health in the general Chinese population: Changes, predictors and psychosocial correlates. *Psychiatry Research*, 293: 113396.

Ellis, W. E., Dumas, T. M., & Forbes, L. M. (2020). Physically isolated but socially connected: Psychological adjustment and stress among adolescents during the initial COVID-19 crisis. *Canadian Journal of Behavioural Science*, 52: 177–187.

Ellis, W. E., Dumas, T. M., & Forbes, L. M. (2020). Physically isolated but socially connected: Psychological adjustment and stress among adolescents during the initial C OVID-19 crisis. *Canadian Journal of Behavioral Science*, 52: 177–187.

Empson, J. (2020, 18th May). What do children think is 'normal'? *The Psychologist*. Retrieved from: https://thepsychologist.bps.org.uk/what-do-children-think-normal

Frey, M., Obermeier, V., von Kries, R., & Schulte-Körne, G. (2020). Age and sex specific incidence for depression from early childhood to adolescence: A 13-year longitudinal analysis of German health insurance data. *Journal of Psychiatric Research*, 129: 17–23.

Gao, J., Zheng, P., Jia, Y., Chen, H., Mao, Y., Chen, S., Wang, Y., Fu, H., & Dai, J. (2020). Mental health problems and social media exposure during COVID-19 outbreak. *PLoS ONE*, 15: e0231924.

Ghosh, R., Dubey, M. J., Chatterjee, S., & Dubey, S. (2020). Impact of COVID-19 on children: Special focus on the psychosocial aspect. *Minerva Pediatrica*, 72: 226–235.

Guessoum, S. B., Lachal, J., Radjack, R., Carrestier, E., Minassian, S., Benoit, L., & Moro, M. R. (2020). Adolescent psychiatric disorders during the covid-19 pandemic and lockdown. *Psychiatry Research*, 291: 113264.

Hrusak, O., Kalina, T., Wolf, J., Balduzzi, A., Provenzi, M., Rizzari, C., Rives, S., del Pozo Carlavilla, M., Alonso, M. E. V., Domínguez-Pinilla, N., et al. (2020). Flash survey on severe acute respiratory syndrome coronavirus-2 infections in paediatric patients on anticancer treatment. *European Journal of Cancer*, 132: 11–16.

Jackson C., Mangtani P., & Vynnycky E. (2014b). *Impact of SCHOOL Closures on an Influenza Pandemic: Scientific Evidence Base Review*. London: Department of Health. Retrieved from: https://assets.publishing.service.gov.uk/government/uploads/system/uploads/attachment_data/file/316203/School_Closures_Evidence_review.pdf

Jackson C., Mangtani P., Hawker, J., Olowokure, B., & Vynnychy, E. (2014a) The effects of school closures on influenza outbreaks and pandemics: Systematic review of simulation studies. *PLoS One*, 9. DOI: 10.1371/journal.pone.0097297

Jiao, W. Y., Wang, L. N., Liu, J., Fang, S. F., Jiao, F. Y., Pettoello-Mantovani, M., & Somekh, E. (2020). Behavioral and emotional disorders in children during the COVID-19 epidemic. *Journal of Pediatrics*, 221: 264–266.

Johnson, R. L., Coleman, R. A., Batten, N. H., Hallsworth, D., & Spencer, E. E. (2020). *The Quiet Crisis of PhDs and COVID-19: Reaching the Financial Tipping Point* Durham, NC, USA: Research Square.

Kapetanovic, S., Gurdal, S., Ander, B., & Sobring, E. (2021). Reported changes in adolescent psychosocial functioning during the COVID-19 outbreak. *Adolescents*, 1(1): 10–20.

Larcombe, W., Finch, S., Sore, R., Murray, C. M., Kentish, S., Mulder, R. A., Lee-Stecum, P., Baik, C., Tokatlidis, O., & Williams, D. A. (2014). Prevalence and socio-demographic correlates of psychological distress among students at an Australian university. *Studies in Higher Education*, 41: 1074–1091.

Leary, M. R. (1990). Responses to social exclusion: social anxiety, jealousy, loneliness, depression and low self-esteem. *Journal of Social and Clinical Psychology*, 9(8): 221–229.

Lee, J. (2020). Mental health effect of school closures during COVID-19, *The Lancet*, 4(6): 241. Retrieved from: https://www.thelancet.com/journals/lanchi/article/PIIS2352-4642(20)30109-7/fulltext

Li, X., Fu, P., Fan, C., Zhu, M., & Li, M. (2021). COVID-19 stress and mental health of students in locked-down colleges. *International Journal of Environmental Research and Public Health*, 18(2): 771. https://pubmed.ncbi.nlm.nih.gov/33477595/

Liu, J. J., Bao, Y., Huang, X., Shi, J., & Lu, L. (2020). Mental health considerations for children quarantined because of covid-19. *Lancet Child and Adolescent Health*, 4: 347–349.

Liu, S., Liu, Y., & Liu, Y. (2020). Somatic symptoms and concern regarding COVID-19 among Chinese college and primary school students: A cross-sectional survey. *Psychiatry Research*, 289: 113070.

Liu, X., Luo, W. T., Li, Y., Li, C. N., Hong, Z. S., Chen, H. L., Xiao, F., & Xia, J. Y. (2020). Psychological status and behavior changes of the public during the COVID-19 epidemic in China. *Infectious Diseases of Poverty*, 9: 58. doi: 10.1186/s40249-020-00678-3

Loades, M. E., Chatburn, E., Higson-Sweeney, N., McManus, M. N., Borwick, C., & Crawley, E. (2020). Rapid systematic review: The impact of social isolation and loneliness on the mental health of children and adolescents in the context of COVID-19. *Journal of the American Academy of Child and Adolescent Psychiatry*, 59(11): 1218–1239.e3

Lyons, Z., Wilcox, H., Leung, L., & Dearsley, O. (2020). COVID-19 and the mental well-being of Australian medical students: Impact, concerns and coping strategies used. *Australasian. Psychiatry*, 28: 649–652.

Mackler, J. S., Kelleher, R. T., Shanahan, L., Calkins, S. D., Keane, S. P., & O'Brien, M. (2015). Parenting stress, parental reactions, and externalizing behavior from ages 4 to 10. *Journal of Marriage and the Family*, 77: 388–406.

Mak, I. W. C., Chu, C. M., Pan, P. C., Yiu, M. G. C., & Chan, V. L. (2009). Long-term psychiatric morbidities among SARS survivors. *General Hospital Psychiatry*, 31: 318–326.

Markel H., Lipman H. B., Navarro J. A., et al. (2007). Nonpharmaceutical interventions implemented by US cities during the 1918–1919 influenza pandemic. *JAMA*, 298(6): 644–654.

Muller, L. M., & Goldenberg, G. (2020). *Education in Times of Crisis: The Potential Implications of School Closures for Teachers and Students*. London, UK: Chartered College of Teaching. Retrieved from: https://chartered.college/wp-content/uploads/2020/05/CCTReport150520_FINAL.pdf

Neece, C., McIntyre, L. L., & Fenning, R. (2020). Examining the impact of COVID-19 in ethnically diverse families with young children with intellectual and developmental disabilities. *Journal of Intellectual Disability Research*, 64: 739–749.

Nearchou, F., Flinn, C., Niland, R., Subramaniam, S. S., & Hennessy, E. (2020). Exploring the impact of COVID-19 on mental health outcomes in children and adolescents: A systematic review. *International Journal of Environmental Research and Public Health*, 17(22): 8479. doi: 10.3390/ijerph17228479

New Zealand Ministry of Health (2017). New Zealand influenza pandemic plan: A framework for action. Available at: https://www.health.govt.nz/publication/new-zealand-influenzapandemic-plan-framework-action (accessed 1 May 2020).

Oberle, E., Ji, X. R., Kerai, S., Guhn, M., Schonert-Reichl, K. A., & Gadermann, A. M. (2020). Screen time and extracurricular activities as risk and protective factors for mental health in adolescence: A population-level study. *Preventive Medicine*, 141: 106291.

Oosterhoff, B., Palmer, C. A., Wilson, J., & Shook, N. (2020). Adolescents' motivations to engage in social distancing during the COVID-19 pandemic: Associations with mental and social health. *Journal of Adolescent Health*, 67: 179–185.

Petrosillo, N., Viceconte, G., Ergonul, O., Ippolito, G., & Petersen, E. (2020). COVID-19, SARS and MERS: Are they closely related? *Clinical Microbiology and Infection*, 26: 729–734.

Prince, J. P. (2015). University student counseling and mental health in the United States: Trends and challenges. *Mental Health Prevention*, 3: 5–10.

Public Health England (2014). Pandemic Influenza Response Plan. Retrieved from: https://assets.publishing.service.gov.uk/government/uploads/system/uploads/attachment_data/file/344695/PI_Response_Plan_13_Aug.pdf (accessed 1 May 2020).

Rajmil, L., Hjem, A., Boran, P., Gunnlaugsson, G., Kraus de Camargo, O., & Raman, S. (2021). Impact of lockdown and school closure on children's health and well-being during the first wave of COVID-19: A narrative study. *BMJ Paediatrics Open*, 5(1). Retrieved from: https://bmjpaedsopen.bmj.com/content/5/1/e001043

Rashid H., Ridda I., King C., et al. (2015). Evidence compendium and advice on social distancing and other related measures for response to an influenza pandemic. *Paediatric Respiratory Review*, 16: 119–126.

Reger, M. A., Stanley, I. H., & Joiner, T. E. (2020). Suicide mortality and coronavirus disease 2019 – A perfect storm? *JAMA Psychiatry*. doi: 10.1001/jamapsychiatry.2020.1060

Sanner, C. M., & Neece, C. L. (2018). Parental distress and child behavior problems: Parenting behaviors as mediators. *Journal of Child and Family Studies*, 27: 591–601.

Seçer, İ., & Ulaş, S. (2020). An investigation of the effect of COVID-19 on OCD in youth in the context of emotional reactivity, experiential avoidance, depression and anxiety. *International Journal of Mental Health and Addiction*, 1–14. doi: 10.1007/s11469-020-00322-z

Shackle, S. (2019, 27th September). 'The way universities are run is making us ill': Inside the student mental health crisis. *The Guardian*. Available online: https://www.theguardian.com/society/2019/sep/27/anxiety-mental-breakdowns-depression-uk-students (accessed on 15 January 2021).

Shanahan, L., Steinhoff, A., Bechtiger, L., Murray, A. L., Nivette, A., Hepp, U., Ribeaud, D., & Eisner, M. (2020). Emotional distress in young adults during the COVID-19 pandemic: Evidence of risk and resilience from a longitudinal cohort study. *Psychological Medicine*, 1–10. doi: 10.1017/S003329172000241X

Stallman, H. M. (2010). Psychological distress in university students: A comparison with general population data. *Australian Psychologist*, 45: 249–257.

Stayner, T. (2020, 27th July). The Young Australians Trapped in the Coronavirus Economy's Dire Job Market. *SBS News*. Available online: https://www.sbs.com.au/news/the-young-australians-trapped-in-the-coronavirus-economy-s-dire-job-market (accessed on 15 January 2021).

Thomas, E. (2020). *Coronavirus: Impact on Young People with Mental Health Needs*; London, UK: Young Minds.

Tian, F., Li, H., Tian, S., Yang, J., Shao, J., & Tian, C. (2020). Psychological symptoms of ordinary Chinese citizens based on SCL-90 during the level I emergency response to COVID-19. *Psychiatry Research*, 288: 112992.

Trzebiński, J., Cabański, M., & Czarnecka, J. Z. (2020). Reaction to the COVID-19 pandemic: The influence of meaning in life, life satisfaction, and assumptions on world orderliness and positivity. *Journal of Loss and Trauma*, 25: 544–557.

UNESCO (2020). Global Education Coalition #LearningNeverStops. COVID-19 Education Response. Retrieved from: https://en.unesco.org/covid19/educationresponse/globalcoalition

Verbruggen, L. C., Wang, Y., Armenian, S. H. Ehrhardt, M. J., van der Pal, H. J. H., van Dalen, E. C., van As, J. W., Bardi, E., Baust, K., Berger, C., et al. (2020). Guidance regarding COVID-19 for survivors of childhood, adolescent, and young adult cancer: A statement from the International Late Effects of Childhood Cancer Guideline Harmonization Group. *Pediatric Blood Cancer*, 67: e28702.

Vinall, M. (2020, 27th May). The class of 2020: What it's like to be graduating in Australia Amid Coronavirus. *SBS News*. Available online: https://www.sbs.com.au/news/the-class-of-2020-what-it-s-like-to-be-graduating-in-australia-amid-coronavirus (accessed on 15 January 2021).

Viner, R. M., Russell, S. J., Croker, H., Packer, J., Ward, J., Stansfield, C., Mytton, O., Bonell, C., & Booy, R. (2020). School closure and management practices during coronavirus outbreaks including COVID-19: A rapid systematic review. *Lancet: Child and Adolescent Health*, 4: 397–404.

Viner, R., Russell, S., Saulle, R., Croker, H., Stansfield, C., Packer, J., Nicholls, D., Goldings, L.-A., Bonell, C., Hudson, L., Hope, S., Schwalbe, N., Porgan, A., & Minozzi, S. (2021). Impacts of schools closures on mental and physical health of children and young people: a systematic review. *JAMA Pediatrics*, 176(4): 400–409. doi: 10.1001/jamapediatrics.2021.5840

Wang, G., Zhang, Y., Zhao, J., Zhang, J., & Jiang, F. (2020). Mitigate the effects of home confinement on children during the COVID-19 outbreak. *Lancet*, 395: 945–947.

Wiseman H. (2008). On failed intersubjectivity: Recollections of loneliness experiences in offspring of Holocaust survivors. *American Journal of Orthopsychiatry*, 78(3): 350–358. doi: 10.1037/a0014197.

World Health Organization (WHO) (2020). *Coronavirus Disease (COVID-19)*. Geneva, Switzerland: WHO.

Wu, K. K., Chan, S. K., & Ma, T. M. (2020). Posttraumatic stress, anxiety, and depression in survivors of severe acute respiratory syndrome (SARS). *Journal of Trauma and Stress*, 18: 39–42.

Xie, X., Xue, Q., Zhou, Y., Zhu, K., Liu, Q., Zhang, J., & Song, R. (2020). Mental health status among children in home confinement during the coronavirus disease 2019 outbreak in Hubei Province, China, *JAMA Pediatrics*, 174: 898–900.

Yang, H., Bin, P., & He, A. J. (2020). Opinions from the epicenter: An online survey of university students in Wuhan amidst the COVID-19 outbreak11. *Journal of Chinese Government*, 5: 234–248.

Zhai, Y., & Du, X. (2020). Mental health care for international Chinese students affected by the COVID-19 outbreak. *Lancet Psychiatry*, 7: e22.

Zhou, S. J., Zhang, L. G., Wang, L. L., Guo, Z. C., Wang, J. Q., Chen, J. C., Liu, M., Chen, X., & Chen, J. X. (2020). Prevalence and socio-demographic correlates of psychological health problems in Chinese adolescents during the outbreak of COVID-19. *European Journal of Child and Adolescent Psychiatry*, 29: 749–758.

Chapter 6

Lockdown and Panic Buying Behaviour

As the initial lockdowns were implemented around the world, among the great uncertainties driving public anxiety was whether normal supply chains would cease to operate. If so, how would this affect the supply of food and other household products, especially those associated with hygiene. Many people, anxious that the closure of many businesses might also mean that supermarkets and other retail outlets that remained open might run out of stock led to panic buying with consumers stockpiling food and household products. This behaviour did result in stores running out of specific commodities for temporary periods. As later-in-the-day consumers turned up to find some supermarket shelves were bare, this could have motivated them to behave similarly wherever they could.

Governments attempted to calm down this atmosphere of uncertainty by reassuring people that the supply chains for essential products would remain open and that they would not be affected by lockdown restrictions. As it became clear that SARS-CoV-2 was mainly an airborne disease, physical distancing rules became more acute. This resulted in restricted numbers of customers being permitted to enter specific retail spaces at any one time to ensure that adequate distances were maintained between those shopping. Such restrictions created queues at many stores. Messages encouraging people to stay home also included the advice that shopping trips should be limited in number. The presence of queues meant that many shoppers were encouraged to reduce their number of shopping trips anyway. When they did go shopping, they still stockpiled to some extent because they sought to ensure they had enough supply of specific products to last until the next trip.

One collateral effect of pandemic-related behaviour restrictions, therefore, was panic buying. This chapter will examine the evidence for this behaviour and also consider pandemic-related behaviour data in the wider context of what was already known about panic buying. This behaviour did not begin with the 2020 pandemic. It was known to occur generally during times of crisis or emergency. Communities that perceive a serious threat, possibly caused by a recent event that might be naturally occurring (e.g., an earthquake, a hurricane or tsunami) or man-made (e.g., an act of terrorism,

DOI: 10.4324/9781003274377-6

a war), will often alter their normal behaviour patterns even without government urging (Forbes, 2017; Wen et al., 2019). On top of this, government-imposed restrictions, such as those imposed during the pandemic, could also be expected to create essential product supply concerns.

Panic buying is mostly characterised by consumers purchasing unusually large quantities of products during or following a period of society-wide crisis or disaster. This behaviour tends to be motivated by a perceived threat that some essential commodities will no longer be available or will have limited supply accompanied by significant increases in price. It is therefore behaviour that anticipates future outcomes that will impact directly on people's lives and where there is considerable uncertainty about how long these outcomes will persist (Yoon et al., 2017; Yuen et al., 2020).

This pattern of buying leads to consumers stockpiling specific commodities for themselves by buying many months supply. This behaviour in turn can result in temporary supply problems ad normal supply chains are unable to keep up with the unusual level of demand. This behaviour benefits a few and then also short changes the many who find that they cannot find the commodities most often targeted by panic buyers (Besson, 2020). This behaviour was observed during the early stages of the pandemic (Loxton et al., 2020).

Under these extreme conditions, public fear and anxiety increase. Plenty of stories circulated in the media that panic buying behaviour was a widespread reaction that has been registered in populations around the world as the 2020 COVID-19 pandemic took hold (Arafat et al., 2020c). One example of this phenomenon in relation to buying food, household products and medications was observed in China at the time of the SARS outbreak in 2003 (Ding, 2009). It was seen also in Japan following the earthquake in 2011 (Wei et al., 2011). What occurred in 2020 was panic buying on a greater scale than previously witnessed and this behaviour was driven to a degree by the widespread chatter on social media (Singh & Rakshit, 2020).

There was widespread news coverage of the COVID-19 outbreak, but this was accompanied by a great deal of online discussion that occurred on social media sites that were relatively unknown even in 2003 during the first SARS coronavirus outbreak. News stories reported panic buying episodes for household goods, especially toilet rolls, and this only served to draw more public attention to it (Jones, 2020). This behaviour was reported all around the world (Sim et al., 2020).

One of the reasons for the publicity given to panic buying is that it occurred in developed nations where consumers are accustomed to no shortages of essentials. While there might sometimes be a run on a new product, such as a new technology, when it comes to everyday foodstuffs, medications and household cleaning products, they tend to be readily available throughout the year. The extreme threat that such commodities might not always be available therefore marks an acute change to normal circumstances. Services that entire populations have come to take for granted might not be available.

Public reaction to this state of affairs combines surprise with shock, anger, anxiety and desperation and despair. Major natural disasters and man-made conflicts have previously affected supply chains, but usually in developing countries where they are not always reliable in normal times. However, developed countries can also experience severe shortages, at least for a short time, following a major disaster (Hori & Iwamoto, 2014; Wilkes, 2020).

The last global pandemic on the scale of COVID-19 was the Spanish flu outbreak in 1918–1919. Revisiting the history of events at the time, researchers have shown that some panic buying of medications occurred which led to threats of shortages (Honigsbaum, 2013). The SARS outbreak in China in 2003 led to panic buying of rice, salt, vegetables, vinegar, face masks and medicines (Ding, 2014). This behaviour did not necessarily result in a breakdown of the social order or wider social unrest. In many ways, it was understandable that people would seek to stock up on essentials if they genuinely believed these items might become unavailable for extended periods (Savage, 2019).

In countries such as the United States, government bodies had previously advised the population to maintain a stockpile of two weeks worth of non-perishable food items in the event of an unexpected national emergency (Federal Emergency Management Agency FEMA, 2004). Similar recommendations have been made to national populations in countries such as Japan and New Zealand that are particularly prone to earthquakes (Thomas & Mora, 2014).

Over-purchasing behaviour can vary between consumers and households. Some people are selective hoarders and will stockpile specific commodities. Others will make a wide array of purchases when confronted with a potential shortage of uncertain duration (Hori & Iwamoto, 2014). In terms of what is known about this behaviour, however, there is far more anecdote based on observations of people's behaviour patterns in relation to specific crisis events than there is systematic behavioural science. What has been gleaned from research designed to understand the psychology of panic buying behaviour, it seems that there just be a perception of genuine threat to the individual and their community, which is accompanied by a spike in anxiety and a further perception that some essentials will become scarce. At a time of such overwhelming uncertainty, panic buying, despite being unhelpful in many ways, represents a coping mechanism that gives the individual a sense that they can take back some personal control over events. Finally, individuals observe the behaviour of others and are driven to conform by engaging in similar behaviour themselves (Yeun et al., 2020).

Panic buying might be labelled as irresponsible and selfish, especially, when authorities give out assurances that essential supply chains will continue to operate. Some individuals are more prone to anxiety in situations of threat and uncertainty and such feelings can become so powerful that they drive them to behave in non-typical ways (Lee & Ashton, 2008). Yet, this impulsive response to a crisis can also be tempered by a degree of civic responsibility and future altruistic intentions. One study showed that individuals scoring higher on a personality scale designed to measure honesty and humility admitted to panic buying but then also recognised that this was probably not the best way to act and indicated they would not repeat it (Columbus, 2020).

This response was not found everywhere. An international study of panic buying behaviour covering people from 35 different countries found that some people had stockpiled and intended to do so again if it was necessary. Such people tended to be those who generally sought more order in their lives and were accustomed to being "in control" and who also felt a lot of anxiety about COVID-19 (Garbe et al., 2020).

Theories of Panic Buying

The excessive purchase of certain goods such as foods, personal hygiene and household products as governments threatened to take extreme measures to control the transmission of the new coronavirus was apparently triggered among some people by the belief that the pandemic would impact upon supply chains rendering some everyday products unavailable. Another practical consideration of many was that if they caught the new virus and became seriously ill, they would be physically unable to go out to shop for these items. This behaviour was not confined to one or two countries, but was observed globally. Despite advisories from governments for people not to stockpile these goods, many still went ahead anyway. In common parlance and in many media reports, this behaviour was generically labelled as "panic buying".

Pre-pandemic research into this pattern of behaviour had associated it with psychological disorders. People who hoarded items or who engaged in regular compulsive purchases were identified as suffering from psychological problems and these behaviours were a response to the difficulties with which they had been dealing. Another perspective on this behaviour was that in a time of national emergency, stockpiling goods was an understandable evolutionary response to the threatened scarcity of resources designed to protect self and one's social group or tribe.

It would probably be a gross oversimplification to explain "panic buying" or excessive purchasing during the early stages of the pandemic as manifestations of psychological disorders. It is possible, however, that people that engaged in this behaviour had experienced adversity in the past and the lessons learned from that experience motivated their purchase behaviour during the pandemic.

This behaviour can also give rise to social tensions between those who have stockpiled and those that have arrived too late to do so. Consumers confronted with empty shelves might be tempted to vent any frustrations and irritation they experience on those still leaving the retail setting with over-full trolleys. Of course, stockpilers have got to be physically and financially able to indulge in this excessive behaviour. There will be others unable to do this because they lack those abilities or resources. Hence, this behaviour serves to highlight discrepancies between the "haves" and the "have nots". Some stockpilers might buy on behalf of others to whom they provide support. So even among the less able to indulge, there will be a further divide between those with and without social support networks. Scratching beneath the surface of this behaviour therefore it is possible to uncover a range of tensions between social groups that have been defined by it (Rajkumar, 2021).

In seeking explanations for panic buying, psychologists and health scientists have explored specific models that have attempted to outline key psychological factors that underpin it or drive it forward. The health belief model is one such theoretical framework that has been extensively tested. It embraces a number of component variables that include whether individuals perceive themselves as susceptible to side-effects of a particular health-related crisis; their assessment of the severity of the crisis and its impact; what they expect to happen next; a search for ideas about how to respond; and then their inner-belief that they are capable of doing something about the uncertain situation in which they find themselves (Sharifikia et al., 2019; Tong et al., 2020; Al-Sabbagh et al., 2021).

In relation then to essential items, individuals will develop perceptions of the probability that they might become scarce during the crisis. The outcome of this assessment in turn will lead them to make specific behavioural choices (i.e., whether to stockpile specific items) and motivate their endeavours to achieve this outcome (Aval et al., 2019, 2021; Arafat et al., 2021).

The health belief model has generally been used to investigate the steps people might take to protect themselves from a health threat, rather than to understand their consumer behaviour. Yet, these two things were interconnected in the 2020 pandemic. People formulated beliefs about the availability of specific commodities during the pandemic and also about their own probability of succumbing to COVID-19. Uncertainty about the consequences of personal infection then fed into calculations about how this might affect their own efficacy not just in protecting themselves but also in being able to show for essentials. When perceived self-efficacy takes a tumble, one response is anxiety (Purzer, 2011). People then worry about whether they will be able to look after themselves and their families. This uncomfortable psychological state will motivate some people to take emergency steps such as stockpiling of commodities while they can. This means doing so while the commodities are available and also while they are fit enough to go and collect them.

Other processes then feed into this psychological process. In a crisis setting, people become more acutely mentally attuned to the latest developments through interpersonal communications, which these days can occur online as well as offline and by monitoring the mass media. They pick up cues about changes to the severity of the ongoing crisis and how it is impacting upon the availability of essential commodities and how it might be changing risks of their own infection. Some people will feel more confident than others about being able to cope with the crisis and to obtain essentials for themselves and their dependents.

Perceptions of the scarcity of specific items and news of tighter restrictions on behaviour as infection rates increase will motivate more immediate coping responses. Panic buying will be motivated for commodities that are believed to be in short supply or for which supply chains could be under threat (Gupta, 2013). The more severe the impact of the crisis on supply chains is perceived to be, the greater the amount of stockpiling behaviour that can be expected (Teubner & Graul, 2020). The drive to buy extra, over and above normal shopping behaviour, will also be driven by the heightened personal risk of infection perceptions that will in turn lead the individual to be anxious about reduced self-efficacy, that is, in the context of COVID-19, becoming too ill themselves to provide for their household (Gupta & Gentry, 2019). Exaggerated conspiracy theories about shortages and about restrictions can become especially powerful behaviour influencers at such times (Brehm, 1966; Suri et al., 2007; Arafat et al., 2021).

Consumer marketing research has indicated that people's perceptions of commodity scarcity can be shaped by feelings of loss of control over circumstances that influence normal consumer behaviour and these feelings, in turn, can trigger anxiety responses coupled with feeling insecure in a setting in which normal service stability has been disrupted (Bonneux & Van Damme, 2006; Hendrix & Brinkman, 2013; Shou et al., 2013). Individuals' own feelings about the possible scarcity of commodities will also be influenced by the perceptions of other people's reactions to this situation.

Evidence was found from historical pandemics that false stories about commodity shortages found their way into popular circulation through extant media and interpersonal gossip that also motivated some people to panic buy. This phenomenon was witnessed during the 1918–1920 Spanish Flu pandemic (Freckelton, 2020). Narratives about scarcity became prevalent during the early phases of the pandemic both before lockdown as well as during it. While news reports simply reported on events that had begun to occur, the attention given to those events drew them to the attention of a wider population and triggered ideas about behaving similarly (Schell, 1997; Dholakia, 2020; Wilkens, 2020).

In some ways, panic buying behaviour represents a primitive response based on a deep-seated need to safeguard providing for our basic, biological needs such as food, a safe home and medication. Normally, these needs are not uppermost in most consumers' minds because supply chains are not normally perceived to be under threat. During the COVID-19 pandemic, however, an unprecedented state of affairs evolved (at least for most people around the world) which caused their consumer judgments to shift in the realisation that normal supply could not be taken for granted (Dodgson, 2021). This behaviour is not driven exclusively by blind panic – which might be defined as an impulsive response. It can also derive from a more strategic approach to taking back control during uncertain times (Arafat et al., 2021). It can also be shaped still further by an absence of confidence in the authorities to deliver on promises to maintain supply chains (Bonneux & Van Damme, 2006).

Perceived scarcity can be influenced not just by public perceptions of supply chain continuity and the buying patterns of other people but also by the judgments people made about the pandemic itself and the degree to which their own lives might be put under threat by it. Fear of contracting the virus, with initial uncertainty about the severity of any illness they suffer, could cause doubts to creep into people's thoughts about how well they might be able to cope with the restrictions introduced by their government and to take care of those dependent upon them.

As earlier chapters have shown, anxiety levels among people, young and old, were elevated during the pandemic and, in some cases, triggered more serious mental health problems (Mamun et al., 2020a, 2020c; Dsouza et al., 2020). Such anxieties stem from exaggerated risk perceptions, but feedback into them. These thoughts and feelings could also cause heightened tensions at home with family members who were also struggling to cope with their own fears (Griffiths & Mamun, 2020; Mamun et al., 2020b).

Public behaviour during the 2020 pandemic was driven by uncertainty concerning how long the pandemic and government restrictions would persist and therefore for how long normal life would have to be put on hold. What was known then, from pre-pandemic research, was that fear can drive panic buying behaviour. Assuming that panic buying was based on false assumptions about disrupted supply chains, it tends to persist for one to two weeks before consumer behaviour settles down into a calmer pattern. Initially, however, it tends to be the most fearful who initiate such behaviour and it can then spread like a contagion with many others joining.

During the early phase of the 2020 pandemic, one commodity on which there was a panic run of stockpiling behaviour was toilet rolls. This commodity is closely associated with personal hygiene and the removal of material that can trigger disgust reactions. When people are frightened of infection, they become more acutely tuned to removing anything from their immediate environment that causes disgust. Any threat to being able to heightened diligence in this context becomes a threat in its own right and in this case drove those most anxious to buy up larger quantities of toilet paper than they would usually (Taylor, 2021).

Research conducted in Singapore before the onset of the circuit breaker the government introduced to halt the spread of the coronavirus showed evidence of panic buying and the relevance of the health belief model in explaining this behaviour (Chua et al., 2020). Data obtained from over 500 Singaporean consumers showed that their perceptions of the probable scarcity of certain essentials because of supply chain problems and then of their own susceptibility to become infected, about the severity of any illness they might experience and how well they might recover all played a part in motivating panic behaviour together with their observations of what people around were doing and the degree to which they felt they were taking back control through stockpiling specific commodities. Panic buying was tempered mostly by feelings of regret upon learning that this behaviour left others, whose needs were perhaps greater than their own, devoid of certain essentials because they were no longer available – at least in the short term (Chua et al., 2020).

A broader review of relevant research evidence confirmed that among the main psychological causes of panic buying were perceived scarcity of products (even when supply chains were not disrupted), their perceived vulnerability or susceptibility to infection, and more general fear of the unknown, and the need to find coping behaviours that could alleviate their anxieties. In the Internet era, social media sites served as echo chambers that magnified these concerns through online chatter that was often littered with half-truths and conspiracy theories (Yuen et al., 2020).

Even though governments can issue assurances to their citizens that essential goods and supplies will not be disrupted by a public health emergency, some people will distrust these messages because they do not trust the government. Observing other people engage in panic buying or turning up to stores to find empty shelves represents powerful evidence that undermines the veracity government promises that supplies of essentials will not be affected and then feeds more behaviour of this kind (Neelamegham & Jain, 1999; Rao et al., 2001; Salmon et al., 2015).

Such copy-cat behaviour will become even more pronounced when individuals witness members of their own family or neighbours and friends engage in panic buying (Neem, 2020). The sharing of images of panic buying episodes and their aftermath (i.e., empty shelves in retail outlets) only serve to cultivate a more widespread climate of uncertainty and panic. During times of great uncertainty and widespread anxiety about personal health and safety, people may be driven to behave in extraordinary ways (Alchin, 2020; Arafat et al., 2020a, 2020b, 2020c; Jezewska-Zychowicz et al., 2020; Laato et al., 2020; Yuen et al., 2020). This extreme behaviour may be especially likely to occur in communities where people are generally risk averse and prefer certainty and control (Kim & Lwin, 2020; Naeem, 2020).

The pandemic caused governments around the world to use extreme public behaviour control measures in the absence of pharmacological interventions and these restrictions had profound economic and psychological effects on people. Dramatic loss of income, social isolation arising from required and, in some locations, enforced stay-at-home measures, and general uncertainty about the future created great stress that resulted in fear and anxiety and many which in a some led to more severe mental health problems. It is therefore understandable that many people behaved uncharacteristically when some of their basic needs came under threat or at least seemed to be (Bentall et al., 2021).

Normal analytical processing and rationale thought could be overwhelmed by fear. Even with the authorities offering whatever assurances they could, the wholescale closure of much of society signalled that there was a major crisis at hand and the threat to the public was severe and very real. Even in socially stable countries such as the Republic of Ireland and the United Kingdom, evidence emerged during the early part of the pandemic that consumer behaviour patterns changed dramatically at the first sign that normal service might be disrupted. The research found that most people (around three-quarters) interviewed about their shopping habits in these two countries admitted to some level of panic buying or stockpiling of specific commodities, mostly foodstuffs and regularly consumed household products (Bentall et al., 2021).

This behaviour was most likely to be observed in households with greater incomes, where there were children, where there was greater anxiety about the pandemic and more distrust of the authorities and of people in general. Over-purchasing was not restricted to one or two products, but tended to extend across a range of products in both Ireland and the United Kingdom.

Measuring Panic Buying

As we have seen, panic buying is linked back to perceptions about product supply but also to perceptions about personal threats caused by a public health crisis involving a new and highly infectious virus. Some researchers have tried to define panic buying behaviour as an aspect of human personality and have examined its links to other personality characteristics and behavioural patterns. The eventual aim has been to develop a psychological test that can measure an individual's propensity to engage in panic buying behaviour.

Not surprisingly, this psychological attribute was found to be related to how people perceive risk, whether they often display impulse buying, their need to control circumstances that present great uncertainty, and their belief that they can exert personal control. Fear and anxiety can be powerful drives of panic buying which means that people more prone to develop anxiety symptoms across a range of social settings might be more likely also to engage in panic buying. As noted earlier, however, the likelihood of panic buying among many can be triggered b the few who do it first. Early panic buyers can set the scene for others to follow (Lins & Aquino, 2020).

Despite what has been learned about the role of anxiety in driving panic buying, further evidence has revealed that there are other psychological dynamics at play. Women tended to display more fear of COVID-19 than did men (Bitan et al., 2020; Broche-Perez et al., 2020; Sakib et al., 2020; Zolotov et al., 2020). Yet men engaged in panic buying to a greater extent than did women (Lins & Aquino, 2020). While men may have been less worried about COVID-19 than women, they were more concerned about disrupted supply chains in respect of essential commodities and felt a stronger urge to do something to take control of this situation (Clemens et al., 2020).

Beliefs, Personality and Panic Buying

Interestingly, despite the prevalence of panic buying and the stockpiling of specific products such as toilet paper, analysis of chatter on sites such as Twitter revealed that there was also widespread dismay at this behaviour. Although some tweets took a somewhat humorous twist about this behaviour, there were many that were highly critical of it. Toilet paper hoarding by a few had deprived many of an essential product (Leung et al., 2021).

Another behavioural model that was used to explain panic buying was the theory of planned behaviour. This theory posited that behaviour patterns can be changed through persuasive messages provided they created favourably attitudes towards the behaviour, cultivate beliefs that behaviour change will make the right kind of difference and perceptions that other people are doing the same, while also encouraging people to think that the behaviour change is within their capabilities.

With regard to panic buying, therefore, if people believe that this is something they must do for good reasons and see others already doing it, and regard the behaviour as within their scope, they will probably conform to others and engage in this kind of behaviour as well. If other people stockpile toilet rolls in the belief that supply of them could run out soon and stockpiling remains possible with the supply remaining, then others will follow suit. Some evidence of this psychological dynamic was found in relation to panic buying in Germany, where it was also explained in terms of reducing the frequency of shopping trips in a climate in which everyone was encouraged to restrict such trips and stay at home (Lehberger et al., 2021).

Further research among consumers in Denmark and the United Kingdom also found that panic buying behaviour was related to specific personality types. People scoring higher on Extraversion and Neuroticism and lower on Conscientiousness and Openness to Experience were more likely to display commodity stockpiling behaviour. In addition, the perception by people that their government could be doing more to manage the pandemic was also associated with a greater propensity to stockpile (Dammeyer, 2020).

Closing Observations

During the early stages of the pandemic, some people became concerned that their government's pandemic-related restrictions would threaten their ability to obtain everyday consumables and especially foodstuffs and household cleaning products. Many retail outlets were compulsorily closed. Although major supermarkets, general stores and pharmacies remained open for business, social distancing rules meant the introduction of tight controls over how many people could enter a store at one time. Further stories surfaced that supply chains would be disrupted resulting in product shortages in supermarkets as manufacturers and delivery firms operated with reduced capacity.

One consequence of these perceived threats was that, for a limited period, shoppers rushed out to supermarkets and emptied the shelves to stockpile far more goods than they would normally purchase. Such behaviour was not unknown during pandemics. As the evidence reviewed in this chapter indicated, panic buying behaviour was observed 100 years earlier during the 1918 Spanish flu pandemic. Further evidence showed that this behaviour occurred among consumers in many different parts of the world.

In trying to explain this behaviour, some researchers of the phenomenon described it as a "primitive" response whereby people become motivated by taking care of their base biological and security needs during times of crisis, when during normal times these needs would be automatically taken care of. Others explained it in terms of people seeking ways to take back some personal control over their lives during a period of great uncertainty.

Governments tried to reassure their citizens that there really was no need to stockpile because major supply chains of everyday commodities, and especially of food, would be unaffected by pandemic-related restrictions. Many consumers chose not to believe this and their hoarding behaviour continued anyway. The result was that latecomers often found shelves empty and were unable therefore to obtain essential products straight away. This behaviour, of course, could have created a broader climate of hoarding as initial "latecomers" in turn may have been motivated to change their shopping habits in order not to lose out in the future.

Over time, the maintenance of supply chains meant that consumers gained reassurance that there would not be shortages caused by supply failures. Nonetheless, not everyone trusted the messages from their governments that normal levels of supply of everyday essentials would be maintained during the pandemic. Indeed, it was the panic buying of consumers themselves that caused temporary problems with supply in the days leading up to the first lockdowns. Further evidence emerged that earlier experiences of panic buying created long-term residual anxiety about future possible buying episodes, especially during holiday seasons such as Christmas. One poll in October 2021 showed that three-quarters of British people (75%) worried that panic buying would disrupt Christmas far outnumbering those concerned about catching COVID-19 and having to socially isolate (54%) (Williams & Millard, 2021). Fortunately, earlier episodes generally showed that this pattern of behaviour was short-lived in most places where it had occurred.

References

Alchin, D. (2020). Gone with the wind. *Australasian Psychiatry*, 28: 636–638.

Al-Sabbagh, M. Q., Al-Ani, A., Mafrachi, B., Siyam, A., Isleem, U., Massad, F. I., Alsabbagh, Q., & Abufaraj, M. (2021). Predictors of adherence with home quarantine during COVID-19 crisis: The case of health belief model. *Psychology of Health and Medicine*, 27(1): 215–227.

Amblee, N., & Bui, T. (2011). Harnessing the influence of social proof in online shopping: The effect of electronic word of mouth on sales of digital micro-products. *International. Journal of Electronic Commerce*, 16: 91–114.

Aquino S. D., Natividade J. C., & Lins S. L. B. (2020). Validity evidences of the buying impulsiveness scale in the Brazilian context. *Psico-USF*, 25(1): 15–25.

Arafat, S. Y., Kar, S. K., Marthoenis, M., Sharma, P., Apu, E. H., & Kabir, R. (2020a). Psychological underpinning of panic buying during pandemic (COVID-19). *Psychiatry Research*, 289: 113061.

Arafat, S., Kar, S. K., Menon, V., Alradie-Mohamed, A., Mukherjee, S., Kaliamoorthy, C., & Kabir, R. (2020b). Responsible factors of panic buying: An observation from online media reports. *Frontiers of Public Health*, 2020(8): 747.

Arafat, S. Y. M., Kar, S. K., Menon, V., Kaliamoorthy, C., Mukherjee, S., Alradie-Mohamed, A., Sharma, P., Marthoenis, M., & Kabir, R. (2020c). Panic buying: An insight from the content analysis of media reports during COVID-19 pandemic. *Neurology, Psychiatry and Brain Research*, 37: 100–103. 10.1016/j.npbr.2020.07.002

Arafat, S., Yuen, K., Menon, V., Shoib, S., & Ahmad, A. (2021). Panic buying in Bangladesh: An exploration of media reports. *Frontiers in Psychiatry*, 11: 628393.

Aval, M. K., Ansari-Moghadam, A. R., & Masoudy, G. (2019). Educational intervention based on Health Belief Model of the adoption of preventive behaviours of Crimean-Congo haemorrhagic fever in ranchers. *Health Scope*, 8: 6.

Bentall, R. P., Lloyd, A., Bennett, K., McKay, R., Mason, L., Muprhy, J., McBride,O., Hartman, T. K., Gibson-Miller, J., Levita, L., Martinez, A. P., Stocks, T. V. A., Butter, S., Vallieres, F., Hyland, P., Karatzias, T., & Shevlin, M. (2021). Pandemic buying: Testing a psychological model of over-purchasing and panic buying using data from the United Kingdom and the republic of Ireland during the early phase of the COVID-19 pandemic, *PLoS ONE*, 16(1): e0246339. Doi: 10.1371/journal.pone.0246339

Besson, E. K. (2020). COVID-19 (Coronavirus): Panic Buying and Its Impact on Global Health Supply Chains. World Bank. Retrieved from: https://blogs. worldbank.org/health/covid-19-coronavirus-panic-buying-and-its-impact-global-health-supply-chains (accessed on 14 June 2020).

Bitan, D. T., Grossman-Giron, A., Bloch, Y., Mayer, Y., Shiffman, N., & Mendlovic S. (2020). Fear of COVID-19 scale: Psychometric characteristics, reliability and validity in the Israeli population. *Psychiatric Research*, 289(1–5): 113100.

Bonneux, L., & Van Damme, W. (2006). An iatrogenic pandemic of panic. *BMJ*, 332: 786–788.

Brehm, J. W. (1966). *A Theory of Psychological Reactance*. Cambridge, MA, USA: Academic Press.

Broche-Pérez Y., Fernández-Fleites Z., Jiménez-Puig E., Fernández-Castillo E., & Rodríguez-Martin B. C. (2020). Gender and fear of COVID-19 in a Cuban population sample. *International Journal of Mental Health and Addiction*, 1–9. doi: 10.1007/s11469-020-00343-8 [E-publication ahead of print].

Carpenter, C. J. (2010). A meta-analysis of the effectiveness of health belief model variables in predicting behaviour. *Health Communication*, 25: 661–669.

Chua, G., Yuen, K. F., Wang, K., & Wong, Y. D. (2020). The determinants of panic buying during COVID-19. *International Journal of Environmental Research and Public Health*, 18(6): 3247. Doi: 10.3390/ijerph18063247

Clemens, K. S., Matkovic, J., Faasse, K., & Geers A. L. (2020). Determinants of safety-focused product purchasing in the United States at the beginning of the global COVID-19 pandemic. *Safety Science*, 130: 104894.

Columbus S. (2020). Who hoards? Honesty-humility and behavioural responses to the 2019/20 coronavirus pandemic. *PsyArXiv [Preprint]*. Available from https://psyarxiv.com/8e62v/

Dammeyer, J. (2020). An explorative study of the individual differences associated with consumer stockpiling during the early stages of the 2020 coronavirus outbreak in Europe. *Personality and Individual Differences*, 167: 110263. doi: 10.1016/j.paid.2020.110263

Dholakia, U. (2020). Why Are We Panic Buying during the Coronavirus Pandemic. Available online: https://www.sandiegouniontribune.com/news/health/story/2020-03-22/hoard-fear-panic-buying-psychology

Ding, H. (2009). Rhetorics of alternative media in an emerging epidemic: SARS, censorship, and extra-institutional risk communication. *Technical Communications Quarterly*, 18(4): 327–350.

Ding. H. (2014). *Rhetoric of a Global Epidemic: Transcultural Communication about SARS*. Carbondale, Ill: Southern Illinois Press.

Ditto, P. H., & Jemmott, J. B. (1989). From rarity to evaluative extremity: Effects of prevalence information on evaluations of positive and negative characteristics. *Journal of Personality and Social Psychology*, 57: 16–26.

Dodgson, L. A. (2021). Human behaviour expert explains 4 psychological reasons why people are panic buying items in bulk during the coronavirus pandemic. Retrieved from: https://www.yahoo.com/news/human-behavior-expert-explains-4-123500438.html?nhp=1

Dsouza, D. D., Quadros, S., Hyderabadwala, Z. J., & Mamun, M. A. (2020). Aggregated COVID-19 suicide incidences in India: Fear of COVID-19 infection is the prominent causative factor. *Psychiatry Research*, 290: 113145.

Federal Emergency Management Agency [FEMA]. (2004). *Food and water in an emergency*. Jessup, MD: FEMA. Available from: https://www.fema.gov/pdf/library/f&web

Forbes, S. L. (2017). Post-disaster consumption: Analysis from the 2011 Christchurch earthquake. *International Review of Retail, Distribution and Consumer Research*, 27: 28–42. doi: 10.1080/09593969.2016.1247010

Freckelton, I. (2020). COVID-19: Fear, quackery, false representations and the law. *International Journal of Law and Psychiatry*, 72: 101611. Doi: 10.1016/j.jilp.2020. 101611

Garbe, L., Rau, R., & Toppe T. (2020). Influence of perceived threat of Covid-19 and HEXACO personality traits on toilet paper stockpiling. *PloS One*, 15: e0234232. pmid:32530911.

Griffiths, M. D., & Mamun, M. A. (2020). COVID-19 suicidal behaviour among couples and suicide pacts: Case study evidence from press reports. *Psychiatry Research*, 289: 113105.

Gupta, S. (2013). *The Psychological Effects of Perceived Scarcity on Consumers' Buying Behaviour*. Ph.D. Dissertation, CA, USA: University of Nebraska, Lincoln.

Gupta, S., & Gentry, J. W. (2016). The behavioural responses to perceived scarcity – the case of fast fashion. *International Review of Retail Distribution Research*, 26: 260–271.

Gupta, S., & Gentry, J. W. (2019). 'Should I Buy, Hoard, or Hide?' –Consumers' responses to perceived scarcity. *International Review of Retail Distribution Research*, 29: 178–197.

Hendrix, C., & Brinkman, H.-J. (2013). Food insecurity and conflict dynamics: Causal linkages and complex feedbacks. *Stability: The International Journal of Security and Development*, 2: 26. Retrieved from: https://www.stabilityjournal. org/articles/10.5334/sta.bm/?utm_source=TrendMD&utm_medium=cpc&utm_ campaign=Stability_TrendMD_1

Honigsbaum, M. (2013). Regulating the 1918–19 pandemic: Flu, stoicism and the Northcliffe press. *Medical History*, 57: 165–185.

Hori, M., & Iwamoto K. (2014). The run on daily foods and goods after the 2011 Tohoku earthquake. *The Japanese Political Economy*, 40: 69–113.

Jezewska-Zychowicz, M., Plichta, M., & Królak, M. (2020). Consumers' fears re-garding food availability and purchasing behaviours during the COVID-19 pandemic: The importance of trust and perceived stress. *Nutrients*, 12: 2852.

Jolly, W. (2020). New data shows massive increases – and decreases – in consumer spending due to COVID-19. *Savings.com.au [Internet]*. 24th March. Retrieved from: https://www.savings.com.au/credit-cards/new-data-shows-massive-increases-and-decreases-in-consumer-spending-due-to-covid-19

Jones, L. (2020 March 26th). What's behind the great toilet roll grab? *BBC News*. Retrieved from https://www.bbc.co.uk/news/business-52040532

Kim, H. K., & Lwin, M. O. (2020). Cultural determinants of cancer fatalism and cancer prevention behaviours among Asians in Singapore. *Health Communication*, 6(8): 940–949. doi: 10.1080/10410236.2020.1724636

Laato, S., Islam, A. N., Farooq, A., & Dhir, A. (2020). Unusual purchasing beha-viour during the early stages of the COVID-19 pandemic: The stimulus-organism-response approach. *Journal of Retailing and Consumer Services*, 57: 102224.

Lee, K., & Ashton, M. C. (2008). The HEXACO personality factors in the in-digenous personality lexicons of English and 11 other languages. *Journal of Personality*, 76: 1001–1054.

Lee S. H., & Workman J. E. (2015). Compulsive buying and branding phenomena. *Journal of Open Innovation Technology Market and Complexity*, 1(1): 3. 10. 1186/s40852-015-0004-x

Lehberger, M., Kleih, A.-K., & Sparke, K. (2021). Panic buying in times of coronavirus (COVID-19): Extending the theory of planned behavior to understand the stockpiling of nonperishable food in Germany. *Appetite*, 161: 105118.doi: 10.1016/j.appetite.2021.105118

Leung, J., Chung, J. Y. C., Tisdale, C., Chiu, V., Lim, C. C. W., & Chan, G. (2021). Anxiety and panic buying behaviour during COVID-19 pandemic – A qualitative analysis of toilet paper hoarding contents on Twitter. *International Journal of Environmental Research and Public Health*, 18(3): 1127. doi: 10.3390/ijerph18031127

Lins, S., & Aquino, S. (2020). Development and initial psychometric properties of a panic buying scale during COVID-19 pandemic. *Heliyon*, 6(9): E04746. doi: 10.1016/j.helyion.2020.e04746

Loxton, M., Truskett, R., Scarf, B., Sindone, L., Baldry, G., & Zhao, Y. (2020). Consumer behaviour during crises: Preliminary research on how coronavirus has manifested consumer panic buying, herd mentality, changing discretionary spending and the role of the media in influencing behaviour. *Journal of Risk and Financial Management*, 13(8): 166, 10.3390/jrfm13080166

Mamun, M. A., Bodrud-Doza, M., & Griffiths, M. D. (2020a). Hospital suicide due to non-treatment by healthcare staff fearing COVID-19 infection in Bangladesh? *Asian Journal of Psychiatry*, 54: 102295

Mamun, M. A., Chandrima, R. M., & Griffiths, M. D. (2020b). Mother and son suicide pact due to COVID-19-related online learning issues in Bangladesh: An unusual case report. *International Journal of Mental Health and Addiction*, 1–4. doi: 10.1007/s11469-020-00362-5

Mamun, M. A., Siddique, A. B., Sikder, M. T., & Griffiths, M. D. (2020c). Student suicide risk and gender: A retrospective study from Bangladeshi press reports. *International. Journal of Mental Health and Addiction*, 1–8. 10.1007/s11469-02 0-00267-3

Markus, H. R., & Schwartz, B. (2010). Does choice mean freedom and well-being? *Journal of Consumer Research*, 37: 344–355.

Naeem, M. (2020). Do social media platforms develop consumer panic buying during the fear of Covid-19 pandemic. *Journal of Retailing and Consumer Services*, 58: 102226.

Neelamegham, R., & Jain, D. (1999). Consumer choice process for experience goods: An econometric model and analysis. Journal of Marketing Research, 36, 373–386.

O'Connell M., de Paula A., & Smith K. (2020). *Preparing for a Pandemic: Spending Dynamics and Panic Buying during the COVID-19 First Wave*. London: Institute for Fiscal Studies. Retrieved from: https://www.ifs.org.uk/publications/15100

Purzer, S. (2011). The relationship between team discourse, self-efficacy, and individual achievement: A sequential mixed-methods study. *Journal of Engineering Education*, 100: 655–679.

Rajkumar, R. P. (2021). A biopsychosocial approach to understanding panic buying: Integrating neurobiological, attachment-based, and social-anthropological perspectives. *Frontiers in Psychiatry*, 12: 652353. doi: 10.3389/fpsyt.2021.652353

Rao, H., Greve, H. R., & Davis, G. F. (2001). Fool's gold: Social proof in the initiation and abandonment of coverage by Wall Street analysts. *Administration Science Quarterly*, 46: 502–526.

Reinstein, D. A., & Snyder, C. M. (2005). The influence of expert reviews on consumer demand for experience goods: A case study of movie critics. *Journal of Indian Economics*, 53: 27–51.

Sakib N., Bhuiyan A., Hossain S., Al Mamun F., Hosen I., Abdullah A. H., Sarker M. A., Mohiuddin M. S., Rayhan I., Hossain M., Sikder M. T., Gozal D., Muhit M., Islam S., Griffiths M. D., Pakpour A. H., & Mamun M. A. (2020). Psychometric validation of the bangla fear of COVID-19 scale: Confirmatory factor analysis and rasch analysis. *International Journal of Mental Health and Addiction*: 1–12.

Salmon, S. J., De Vet, E., Adriaanse, M. A., Fennis, B. M., Veltkamp, M., & De Ridder, D. T. (2015). Social proof in the supermarket: Promoting healthy choices under low self-control conditions. *Food Quality and Preference*, 45: 113–120.

Savage, D. A. (2019). Towards a complex model of disaster behaviour. *Disasters*, 43: 771–798.

Schell, H. (1997). Outburst! A chilling true story about emerging-virus narratives and pandemic social change. *Configurations*, 5: 93–133.

Segal, B., & Podoshen, J. S. (2013). An examination of materialism, conspicuous consumption and gender differences. *International Journal of Consumer Studies*, 37(2): 189–198.

Sharifikia, I., Rohani, C., Estebsari, F., Matbouei, M., Salmani, F., & Hossein-Nejad, A. (2019). Health belief model-based intervention on women's knowledge and perceived beliefs about warning signs of cancer. *Asia-Pacific Journal of Oncology Nursing*, 6(4): 431–439. doi: 10.4103/apjon.apjon_32_19

Sheu J.-B., & Kuo H.-T. (2020). Dual speculative hoarding: A wholesaler-retailer channel behavioural phenomenon behind potential natural hazard threats. *International Journal of Disaster Risk Reduction*, 44: 101430.

Shou, B., Xiong, H., & Shen, X. (2013). Consumer panic buying and quota policy under supply disruptions. *Manufacturing and Services Operations Management*, 6: 1–9.

Sim, K., Chua, H. C., Vieta, E., & Fernandez, G. (2020). The anatomy of panic buying related to the current COVID-19 pandemic. *Psychiatry Research*, 288: 113015. pmid:32315887.

Singh, C. K., & Rakshit, P. (2020). A critical analysis to comprehend panic buying behaviour of Mumbaikar's in COVID-19 era. *Studies in Indian Place Names*, 40(69): 44–51.

Sterman, J. D., & Dogan, G. (2015). "I'm not hoarding, I'm just stocking up before the hoarders get here." Behavioural causes of phantom ordering in supply chains. *Journal of Operational Management*, 15(39–40): 6–22.

Suri, R., Kohli, C., & Monroe, K. B. (2007). The effects of perceived scarcity on consumers' processing of price information. *Journal of the Academy of. Marketing Science*, 35: 89–100.

Taylor, S. (2021). Understanding and managing pandemic-related panic buying. *Journal of Anxiety Disorders*, 78: 102364. doi: 10.1016/j.anxdis.2021.102364

Teubner, T., & Graul, A. (2020). Only one room left! How scarcity cues affect booking intentions on hospitality platforms. *Electronic Commerce Research and Applications*, 39: 100910.

Thomas, J. A., & Mora, J. A. (2014). Community resilience, latent resources and resource scarcity after an earthquake: Is society really three meals away from anarchy? *Natural Hazards*, 74: 477–490.

Tong, K. K., Chen, J. H., Yu, E. W. Y., & Wu, A. M. (2020). Adherence to COVID-19 precautionary measures: Applying the health belief model and generalised social beliefs to a probability community sample. *Applied Psychology: Health and Well-Being*, 12: 1205–1223.

Verdugo, G. B., & Ponce, H. R. (2020). Gender differences in millennial consumers of Latin America associated with conspicuous consumption of new luxury goods. *Global Business Review*, 1–14. doi: 10.1177/0972150920909002

Wei K., Wen-Wu D., & Lin W. (2011). 2011 International Conference on Management Science & Engineering 18th Annual Conference Proceedings. IEEE; Research on emergency information management based on the social network analysis – a case analysis of panic buying of salt; pp. 1302–1310.

Wen, X., Sun, S., Li, L., He, Q., & Tsai, F. S. (2019). Avian influenza-factors affecting consumers' purchase intentions toward poultry products. *International Journal of Environmental Research and Public Health*, 16(21): 4139. doi: 10.3390/ijerph16214139

Wilkens, J. (2020). The San Diego Union-Tribune. Why We Hoard: Fear at Root of Panic Buying, *Psychologists Say*. 2020. Available online: https://www.sandiegouniontribune.com/news/health/story/2020-03-22/hoard-fear-panic-buying-psychology

Wilkes J. (2020). Has there always been panic buying? And when have people panic shopped through history? *History Extra [Internet]*. 7th May 2020. Retrieved from: https://www.historyextra.com/period/20th-century/toilet-paper-shortage-why-do-people-stockpile-panic-buying-history-rationing/

Williams, B., & Millard, H. (2021, 8th October). Panic buying is the public's biggest worry in the run up to Christmas. Ipsos-MORI. Retrieved from: https://www.ipsos.com/ipsos-mori/en-uk/panic-buying-publics-biggest-worry-run-up-to-christmas

Worchel, S., & Brehm, J. W. (1971). Direct and implied social restoration of freedom. *Journal of Personality and Social Psychology*, 18: 294–304.

Yoon, J., Narasimhan, N., & Kim, M. K. (2017). Retailer's sourcing strategy under consumer stockpiling in anticipation of supply disruptions. *International Journal of Production Research*, 56: 3615–3635.

Yuen, K. F., Wang, X., Ma, F., & Li, K. X. (2020). The psychological causes of panic buying following a health crisis. *International Journal of Environmental Research and Public Health*, 17(10): 3513. Doi:10.3390/ijerph17103513

Zheng R., Shou B., & Yang J. (2020). Supply disruption management under consumer panic buying and social learning effects. *Omega*, 101(1): 102238. doi:10.1016/j.omega.2020.102238

Zolotov Y., Reznik A., Bender S., & Isralowitz R. (2020). COVID-19 fear, mental health, and substance use among Israeli university students. *International Journal of Mental Health and Addiction*. 1–7. Retrieved from: https://link.springer.com/article/10.1007/s11469-020-00351-8

Chapter 7

Friendships, Romance and Social and Sexual Relations

As the evidence presented in earlier chapters showed, for some people, pandemic-related restrictions triggered severe psychological reactions that could have an impact on their general health. The side-effects of lockdown extended beyond making people more anxious, stressed or depressed. Behavioural restrictions also interfered with interpersonal relationships. Being confined to home, often because of school and office closures, meant that families were thrown together at times they would normally have been apart. Not everyone had space at home to provide a comfortable work or study environment. Established personal relationships could be put under strain resulting in serious mental health issues for individuals and also sometimes being projected onto others, with seriously harmful consequences. Extreme social isolation also meant that it was virtually impossible for those entering or seeking new relationships to make much headway – except that the main substitute for face-to-face contact was "virtual" contact. With relationships being developed and maintained through physical contact as well as through verbal communication, lockdown placed many under strain or at least required those taking part to adapt to different forms of interaction (Lenzer, 2020).

What became clear as more behavioural scientists started to investigate these issues was that lockdowns might be necessary to control an airborne pandemic, but they could also cause a great deal of harm. Furthermore, this "harm" came in many forms and was not distributed evenly across populations. Some population sub-groups felt the strain more than others. Part of the reason for this variance in psychological damage stemmed from the fact that some people faced a greater risk of falling seriously ill or dying from COVID-19 than did others (Public Health England, 2020). In addition, behavioural restrictions starved many people of the social contact to which they were accustomed. For those who depended on this contact for emotional sustenance, taking it away could have serious psychological consequences for them.

Even though there was evidence that men were more likely to die from the new coronavirus than were women, women tended to have more and

DOI: 10.4324/9781003274377-7

stronger negative psychological experiences associated with the pandemic (Gausman & Langer, 2020). As we will see, later in this book, women were also more likely than men to experience physical violence triggered by the pressures of the lockdown, especially at home (Usher et al., 2020). With schools being closed, and households being placed under additional pressure as parents and carers assumed responsibility for their children's day-to-day educational needs, women bore the brunt of this pressure (Collins et al., 2021). Those from minority sexual orientation groups also experienced increased stress if they had to return home to live with their families to whom they had not disclosed their sexuality or may have felt obliged to play it down or hide it (Jowett, 2020).

Under dramatically introduced restrictions, people's entire social lives were wrenched from under them. Such individuals understandably felt socially isolated. Among these individuals, those happy with their own company coped better than did those for whom regular social contact was critical to their general mental well-being. Social distancing restrictions for many people, however, cultivated feelings of loneliness, especially among those already on their own but in relationships with others from different households (Aarts et al., 2015). Research both before and during the pandemic showed that when opportunities for close social and intimate behaviour are removed from individuals loving on their own, such restrictions can have a serious and sometimes harmful psychological impact which is not exclusive to older people (Hawkley et al., 2003; Levin, 2004; Matthews et al., 2017; Lehmiller et al., 2021; Li & Wang, 2020). In this chapter therefore attention will be turned to the impact of the pandemic and its related restrictions on social behaviour involving new and established relationships.

Importance of Romance

Romantic relationships are not just biologically important in terms of the procreation of the species, they can also enhance our psychological and physical health (Pietromonaco & Beck, 2017, 2019). The introduction of social distancing rules which prohibited many of these romantic and sexual relationships therefore placed many couples under stress on couples (Overall et al., 2020). Couples in an established relationship who did not live together were initially prohibited from seeing each other face-to-face. If they had already been living in the same household before lockdown rules were introduced, they were not affected by this restriction. These restrictions were believed to place these "living part together" under strain and could result in a deterioration in their relationship which included increased conflict between partners (Balzarini et al., 2020).

Lockdown and People's Sex Lives

The lockdown restrictions potentially undermined people's sex lives. This consequence applied not just to sexually involved couples in established relationships when they did not live together, but also individuals with sexually more promiscuous lives who engage in casual sexual liaisons. This has been given the technical term of "sociosexuality" (Simpson & Gangestad, 1991). For some people, this behaviour is unacceptable in general or especially if they have committed to one other person, but for others it is regarded as acceptable and satisfying (French et al., 2019). A propensity to engage in casual sex does not always sit well with being married and more often than not results in marital dissatisfaction (French et al., 2019). Some couples are tolerant of this behaviour however (Rodrigues et al., 2017). For those individuals for whom sociosexuality is important, any enforced prohibition of it removes an activity that might be psychologically beneficial to them (Vrangalova & Ong, 2014). Hence regardless of one's ethical position on this behaviour, for some people its removal under legally enforced behavioural restrictions can have a negative psychological impact on them. This impact might be especially strongly experienced by single people for whom open sexual behaviour is currently part of their normal course of life. Research among gay and bisexual men found that a substantial minority (40%) said they had continued to engage in casual sexual relationships during lockdown (Shilo & Mor, 2020).

Although pandemic restrictions resulted in deprivation of sexual activity for some people, for others it caused a weakening of their sex drive to a point where even though sex was available to them within their household, they did not feel in the mood. Evidence emerged from different parts of the world, not just of young people experiencing a decrease in sexual partners, but also of people across all age groups and relationship types being less sexually active (Li et al., 2020).

While support for a decline in sexual interest emerged among some population sub-groups, among others, reports were found of increased activity. In the United States, around half of people surveyed in one study reported having less sex, but one in five said they had been having more (Lehmiller et al., 2021).

The behavioural restrictions imposed during lockdown had implications for people's personal, sexual and intimate relationships. The severity of these implications will depend upon the nature of the relationship, how well established it is, and the personalities involved. New relationships between partners living in different households will be significantly affected because under some of the more draconian restrictions in which people who do not live together are not allowed to meet face-to-face, these embryonic romances might be ended before they begin. For more established relationships between people who do not officially yet live together, face-to-face contact might be prohibited unless they move in together. Time apart could be difficult to deal with if the relationship has reached a point where both partners expect regular close physical contact. Moving in together prematurely however could also put the relationship under strain that causes it to collapse (BPS, 2020, 30th November).

Digital technologies provide one solution allowing regular virtual "face-to-face" communication that might keep the relationship alive provided the behavioural restrictions do not persist for too long. Once again, the prognosis in terms of eventual outcome will depend upon the status of the relationship and how committed to it each partner is.

The pressures of the pandemic triggered by the anxiety it causes can also place even established relationships under strain. Even when both partners already live together, they may not be accustomed to being with each other all day long. Yet, if both are required to work from home, this will be the outcome. If one partner works from home and the other loses their job, emotional tensions in the household could become even more acute. This could in turn damage the intimacy in the relationship.

Another important coping strategy is to develop regular routines across the week to give structure to everyday life while normality is suspended. This means allocating times to work and times for leisure and entertainment. Time might be assigned to each partner being on their own and then doing things together. Some of the "together" things should involve leaving the house for a joint change of scene. There will be routine shopping trips, unless all provisions are delivered or to take exercise.

The enforced suspension of normal everyday life also gives the partnership an opportunity to reflect on how they might wish to make permanent changes to the way they live their life. It will provide an opportunity for partners to explore doing new things together which could strengthen the relationship by refreshing it.

Even when a couple lived apart and find themselves prohibited from meeting face-to-face in ways that allow them to be intimate with each other, they can explore "being together, apart" as a new relationship format that allows them to put the strength of their relationship to the test. They can still plan to do things together, but remotely. These circumstances will enable them to look at each other and their relationship from a different perspective and evaluate what they really like about it (or not).

Single people were confronted with specific challenges during lockdown periods and other periods when behavioural restrictions meant they still could not hook up with a stranger. For many, the pandemic meant that their sex lives were put on hold. There were still ways in which they could connect with other people virtually, but establishing new physical relationships was largely out of bounds.

The challenges could be equally pronounced for people who lived together in established relationships. Forced to work from home, they might actually find themselves together but also apart as they focused on coming to terms with a new way of working. It was important here for such couples to create opportunities to be together away from their work. This was easier when work was conducted elsewhere outside the home. Once the home became the workplace, the demands on their daily time budget at home changed and such changes could have implications for how much quality time they really spent together. Couples also obtain social sustenance through their friendship groups with which they often engage as a "couple". It was important therefore to keep these connections through regular virtual get-togethers with friends.

A survey by Ipsos-MORI, conducted shortly after the implementation of the first lockdown in March 2020, questioned people across Britain about how the pandemic and lockdown had affected their romantic relationships. In this survey, one in five Britons in relationships (19%) said that they had been arguing more with their partner during the pandemic. Women (25%) were twice as likely as men (12%) to report this kind of behaviour change. The presence of children in the home also led to more reports of arguments than occurred in homes without children (24% vs 16%). Slightly more said they were less often over moe often making plans for the future (24% vs 19%).

Overall, the pandemic seemed to benefit established relationships more often than damage them. More respondents said that they had grown closer to their partner (41%) during the pandemic than grown further apart (10%). This was especially likely among those aged 18–34 (59% vs 17%). Among the older age groups, most (55%) were likely to say their relationship had not changed noticeably during the pandemic, (though more felt it had improved (35%) than got worse (7%) (Beaver et al., 2020, 18th November).

There was some evidence that people in established relationships were arguing more during the pandemic than they had been doing before it. One in five of those questioned by Ipsos-MORI (19%) admitted to this. There was a gender difference in reporting this behaviour with women (25%) being twice as likely as men (12%) to say there had been more arguments with their partner during the pandemic. Couples were also more likely to say they had been arguing more in households with children (24%) than in households with no children (16%). Increased arguing might be linked to the fact that many couples were spending more time together than they would normally (43% said this). As the next chapter will show, arguments can sometimes evolve into full-blown violent altercations in which people can sometimes get seriously hurt.

Turning to more romantic behaviours, the pandemic did not seem to have made much difference to the number of sex couples said they were having. Only a modest minority (15%) said they were having more sex, while a similar proportion (14%) said they were having less. Of those in relationships, it was the youngest aged 18–34 (31%) that were most likely to be more sexually active (double the overall average of 15%). Regardless of whether couples were being more sexual, a substantial proportion (41%) said they had grown closer to their partner since the coronavirus outbreak began. This figure was substantially higher again amongst the young couples aged 18–34 (59%).

In another study of people's sexual activity during the lockdown, soundings were taken from a sample of 800+ adults over one week. Sexual activity was defined as sexual intercourse, masturbation, petting or fondling. Key characteristics most closely associated with continued sexual activity during lockdown were being male, being relatively young and being married or cohabiting (Jacob et al., 2020). The researchers did not measure changes in lockdown sexual activity compared with pre-lockdown levels. A leading United Kingdom pollster, however, surveyed nearly 12,000 British adults and found that they reported a general decrease in sexual activity across all age groups (Nolsoe, 2020). On the evidence provided by these respondents, it seems that social isolation restrictions played a major part in changes to sexual activity. This relationship could be explained not only in terms of reductions in physical opportunities for sex between partners, but also as a consequence of mental and physical health side-effects of lockdown.

When the lockdown was first implemented in Britain in March 2020 indoor face-to-face meetings between people not from the same household were prohibited. Such restrictions presented affected lots of people but were particularly difficult for those entering new romantic relationships or trying to sustain such relationships with individuals they did not live with. Young people were disproportionately affected by these rules.

One survey of young British people, aged 18–32, questioned them about their sex lives before and during the lockdown and found that much of their sexual activity, especially intercourse, had decreased significantly during the lockdown. Around a quarter (26%) stopped this activity completely during the lockdown. This still meant that a substantial proportion continued to maintain a sex life with their partner, with around one-fifth claiming to be more sexually active and one-third saying they were less active (Wignall & McCormack, 2021; Wignall et al., 2021).

Across all people, and not just those who were single, one in five said they had been less sexually active during the pandemic than before it. One in seven (14%) claimed that their sex lives had become significantly less active. A few people (7%) claimed they were having more active sex lives with live-in partners (Nolsoe, 2020, 12th June). There were age differences in these responses. Nearly, four in ten of those aged 18–24 (38%) said they were having less sex than usual (i.e., compared with the six months before lockdown), with eight per cent saying they were having more. Between one in five and one in four of those in the next three older age groups, 25–34 (23%), 35–44 (29%) and 45–54 (20%) said they were having less lockdown sex. These proportions significantly outnumbered those in each of these age groups who said they were more sexually active during lockdown (15%, 11% and 6%, respectively).

Research conducted by the National Surveys of Sexual Attitudes and Lifestyles (Natsal) questioned a large national British sample (6,000+ respondents) online about their sexual behaviour from the start of the first United Kingdom lockdown on 23rd March 2020. The fieldwork took place between the end of July and the middle of August 2020. Evidence emerged that the lockdown had exerted a considerable impact on people's sex lives, with young people and those not already living it their sexual partner being most affected. Although people continued with their sex lives, whether solo or in a partner relationship, there were downward shifts noted in the amount of sex and in how satisfying it was (Mitchell et al., 2020).

Four in ten respondents (38%) reported no sexual contact during the first lockdown, while over half (52%) said they had had sex with a live-in partner and one in ten (10%) claimed to have been intimate with someone from outside their own home. For most of these people, sexual contact was manifest in the form of intimate sexual acts. Intimate contact outside the home was most likely to be reported by those who said they had multiple sexual partners (43%), in gay relationships (20%), the under-25s (18%).

Overall, for over half the sample (55%) the frequency of their sex lives had not changed with lockdown, but more reported having less sex (30%) than more sex (15%). Having less sex was not confined exclusively to those with no regular live-in sexual partner although they were the most likely to report this outcome. Turning then to the quality of their sex lives, most (64%) reported no change, with more saying sex had become less satisfying (20%) than more so (15%) (Pebody, 2021).

An Australian study found that over half (54%) of those surveyed (n = 1,187) said they had less sex during lockdown compared with an equivalent period in 2019. There was a significant drop in those saying they had had sex with casual hook-ups between 2019 and 2020 (31–8%) and slightly fewer singletons reported said they had had lockdown sex with boyfriends/girlfriends during lockdown than the year before (45% versus 42%). Married respondents in contrast said they had been more likely to have sex with their spouse during lockdown than in 2019 (42% versus 35%) (Coombe et al., 2020).

Solo sexual activity reportedly increased among some respondents with one in seven (15%) saying they had been more likely to use sex toys in lockdown than a year earlier and one in four (26%) claiming to have masturbated more often during the lockdown. More respondents said they had used dating apps during lockdown than in 2019 (42% versus 27%). Using these sites specifically to set up virtual dates also increased from 2019 to 2020 (3–17%).

The impact of lockdown and the pandemic on sexual activity varied between different groups of people. There were differences between single people and those who were married or living with their sexual partner.

Research conducted in the UK showed that most people complied with the lockdown restrictions imposed upon the public by the UK government from 23rd March 2020 specifically in the context of dating and sexual behaviour. Researchers confirmed this observation upon questioning a sample of 868 adults online about their sex lives.

At the time of the survey, respondents had been in isolation for an average of nine days. The research found that 40% of respondents had been engaging in sexual activity at least once a week. The highest rates of sexual activity were found among those in a domestic partnership and among younger men who consumed alcohol. In total, 60% of respondents were not engaging in regular sexual activity. In some cases, there were people who felt stressed and anxious about the pandemic and its impact and therefore were not in the mood for sex. There were other cases of individuals who were in a relationship but with someone, they did not live with. The COVID-19 restrictions meant that they were not allowed to meet their romantic partners (Jacob et al., 2020).

A survey introduced earlier found evidence of changes in young adults' sexual desire during the lockdown. It was certainly true that lockdown restrictions had restricted physical opportunities for romantic and sexual partners to get together. Even when they could get together or were already living together, however, the drive for sex weakened among many, especially among women. This was not the case for all sexual partners that lived together, however, with some reporting increased sexual activity. It emerged also that young people whose lives had entered a phase in which they engaged with more than one sexual partner and had causal hook-ups, the impact that lockdown had had on this pattern of behaviour did result in many of these individuals feeling, subjectively at least, less fulfilled and less happy with life. This mood state however did not necessarily translate into a significant increase in health problems (Wignall & McCormack, 2021; Wignall et al., 2021).

From the same research emerged further evidence that men largely hung on to their pre-lockdown sexual desires, with only a non-significant drop, but women were more likely to report a significant decrease in desire during the lockdown. One observation suggested that enforced changes to living arrangements during the lockdown, with adult children returning to the parental home, could have triggered changes in sexual desire, but evidence did not emerge for this phenomenon in this survey (Wignall & McCormack, 2021; Wignall et al., 2021).

Some reviews of evidence found that the COVID-19 pandemic and the associated restrictions on public behaviour deployed by governments in different parts of the world did have various effects on the interpersonal relationships between people and on their sexual relationships in particular. These effects either derived from restrictions that meant that romantic and sexual partners who did not live together could not meet up or from changes to the psychological health of those living together (Ibarra et al., 2020).

A study conducted in Spain when stringent home confinement measures had been put in place in much of the country showed some evidence for decreased sexual activity reported by women. Around seven in ten respondents claimed to have been sexually active and over seven in ten of these were women. These sexually active individuals reported sexual activity an average of just over twice a week. After controlling for differences in sexual activity associated with age, marital or living arrangement status (i.e., partners who lived or did not live together), employment status (in work or unemployed), income level, alcohol consumption and smoking behaviour, there was evidence mostly among women that reported sexual activity showed a statically significant drop once pandemic-related behaviour restrictions had been implemented (López-Bueno et al., 2021).

A British survey (63% women) asked respondents how often, on average, they engaged in sexual activity each week after self-isolation rules had been implemented. As with the Spanish study, the researchers collected data on a range of personal characteristics that could then be statically controlled to isolate the specific effects of lockdown on sexual activity. These details included gender, age, marital status, employment status, income, smoking status, alcohol consumption and mental and physical health, together with any symptoms detected during pandemic-related behavioural restrictions.

During the period of social isolation/social distancing restrictions, four in ten respondents reported sexual activity at least once a week. This activity was greater among males, younger adults, married respondents or those in a live-in domestic partnership, the consumption of alcohol and more days of self-isolation/social distancing. Women, those who were older, not married and did not drink alcohol reported lower levels of sexual activity once lockdown had been implemented (Jacob et al., 2020).

Dating Behaviour

Lockdown and social distancing restrictions have constrained the romantic relationships of many single people. While those living together could continue to enjoy and develop their partnerships, although as we will see, for some prolonged close contact had the opposite effect, for single people all opportunities for direct face-to-face meetings were put in indefinite hold. Dating in intimate settings, holding hands, hugging and kissing were all banned between those who did not live together. Some singletons were, in any case, too afraid to get intimate in the conventional ways for fear of catching COVID-19. Live video calls became the order of the day.

Research by dating agencies detected that fear of COVID extended to a wider fear of dating. Survey findings by big dating companies such as eHarmony found that over one in five 18–34-year-olds felt too anxious to date, even remotely (Butterworth, 2021). Many young people in the late 10s and 20s felt they had suffered a social skills breakdown and close physical contact with another human being made them feel uncomfortable. Yet, other dating applications, such as Tinder, reported an increase in users stating in their biographical profiles that they sought someone they could cuddle and hold hands with (Butterworth, 2021).

Further evidence on the prevalence of sexually transmitted diseases such as gonorrhoea showing that case numbers had increased during 2020 and had reached record levels in England indicated that not everyone had been compliant with lockdown behavioural restrictions. Sites such as Tinder reported upsurges in use of their sites during the early months of the pandemic both in terms of people looking for people and making conversational contact with them. Other dating sites, such as eHarmony, OKCupid and Match, also reported increased business during the pandemic. There were changes happening however. Young people sought richer online communications experiences and this drove a demand for more video links. These are used not just for one-on-one conversations, but also for wider social interactions with virtual groups of people (Shaw, 2020).

Polling among people across Great Britain as the first lockdown was nearing its final stages found that six in ten (60%) of single people said they were not actively dating. They preferred to be alone at that time. It is interesting to note, however, that more than this (67%) said they had gone on no dates at all in the six months before the pandemic. Even the ones that were active daters, nearly half (45%) said they had stopped looking for a new partner completely during the pandemic. While others still sought out new friends, this was mostly done at a distance. One in five (19%) said they were using online dating apps more often and one in ten (9%) said they went on virtual dates (Nolsoe, 2020, 12th June).

There were age differences in dating behaviour patterns. Young adults aged 18–24 (39%) were the least likely across all age groups to say they had stopped dating. Older daters, aged 45–55 years (55%) were most likely to say they had suspended their dating activities. The evidence gathered by this YouGov poll confirmed the reports of dating companies that the use of their services had gone up during the pandemic. A few people, however, had gone back to familiar territory and started re-connecting with former partners (7%). A tiny proportion (1%) flouted lockdown rues and went on physical dates.

Women and Sexual Relationships

The impact of social isolation and distancing restrictions imposed on entire national populations by their governments during the peak infection periods of the pandemic triggered widespread increases in public anxiety and depression. These restrictions also caused frustration which, as we will see later, could sometimes spill over into dysfunctional and destructive behaviour not least among those who lived in close proximity.

Even where live-in relationships found ways of coping with the stress of COVID-19, anxieties did not subside completely and could have an impact on behaviour.

Such behavioural effects included the ways sexual behaviour may have changed during the pandemic. Evidence was found that the restrictive measures of lockdown could influence the sexual function and quality of sex life for women living with a partner. Observational research with sexually active women, mostly aged 28–50, in live-in relationships, found that the number of episodes of sexual intercourse with their partner reduced during the pandemic to around one-third of pre-pandemic levels. The quality of their sex lives was also rated as having deteriorated during the pandemic (Schiavi et al., 2020).

Research emerged that some women, especially those with pre-existing symptoms such as vaginismus derived less pleasure from intercourse despite engaging in treatments designed to reduce their symptoms. One reason given for this was the increased stress and anxiety caused by the pandemic which had rendered sexual interaction as sufferers were unable to relax sufficiently (Ugurlucan et al., 2021).

Men and Sexual Functioning

For some men, the onset of pandemic-related restrictions with related stressors as well as concerns about the new coronavirus itself triggered mental health issues that, for some, became manifest in their sexual performance. The restrictions imposed by governments during the pandemic, which included the closure of many workplaces with job losses or reduced income levels, represented dramatic changes to people's lifestyles and quality of life. These changes might also influence an individuals' general state of health and in turn affect their moods and functioning. Evidence was found from a number of countries around the world that pandemic-related social contact restrictions affected people's sex lives. Much of the attention of research on this subject surveyed either female samples or mixed female-male samples. The sexual activity of heterosexual men attracted much less interest. Yet, what research was carried out with men showed that they were not immune to adverse effects of social distancing and social isolation restrictions.

The outcomes of pandemic impact include reduced sexual activity, decreased satisfaction with own sex life and increased reports of deterioration of relationships with partners. In some cases, however, sex lives were negatively impacted by changes to normal living circumstances, with multiple family members moving in together to maintain regular contact (Cito et al., 2021).

Research in China with a mixed female and male sample showed that over four in ten (44%) reported a decrease in their number of sexual partners during the pandemic and nearly four in ten (37%) reported a fall in frequency of having sex (Li et al., 2020).

Research among Chinese men during the 2020 pandemic found not only that many had less active sex lives but those that did have sexual partners exhibited increased rates of erectile dysfunction and premature ejaculation, which were generally accompanied by higher levels of anxiety and depression (Fang et al., 2021).

Gay Relationships

The pandemic saw the introduction of restrictions of social mixing that potentially undermined the freedom observed in parts of the gay community to engage with many different sexual partners. The onset of HIV/AIDS in the 1980s had caused greater caution among those who were most promiscuous, although for some the protection that was believed to be afforded by wearing condoms reduced the risks. Over time, pharmaceutical treatments have developed that means that acquiring HIV is no longer a death sentence. Research evidence has emerged that over the years before the pandemic, there were signs that men who had sex with other men had reduced their use of condoms. HIV infection levels and deaths from AIDS had been in decline and continued in this vein, but the prevalence of other sexually transmitted diseases had increased as men who had casual sex with other men took fewer physical precautions such as condom wearing. Among men in steady relationships with other men, condom use did not change very much over time (Van Bilsen et al., 2021).

The behavioural restrictions introduced by many countries to slow the spread of COVID-19 focused on limiting social interactions. Inevitably, such interventions could be expected to have an impact on physically intimate liaisons outside of steady live-in relationships. Research among men who had sex with other men indicated that while some observed increased caution in their sexual practices, this did not always extend to total avoidance of linking up with new sexual partners (Lopez de Sousa et al., 2021).

Evidence emerged that men who identified as gay, bisexual or as men who had sex with other men exhibited increased caution about sexual partners during the pandemic. Although this was not true for everyone in this community, there were signs of greater monogamy and revised sexual practices. Walsh et al. (2021) interviewed a sample of over 200 men in the United States about their sexual practices and found that one in seven (15%) said they had changed, developed or ended specific agreements they had reached with other men about sexual behaviour at this time.

In the great majority of these cases, the pandemic emerged consistently as a factor that influenced their decisions. Changed sexual practices included having fewer sexual partners and changed the way they had sex compared with the three months pre-pandemic. Even those with a primary partner reported some changes to their sexual behaviour that might usually be associated with caution against sexually transmitted diseases. Others restricted their decisions to change sexual practices to partners outside their main relationship. These changed behaviour patterns were often explained in terms of prevention of COVID-19 transmission and also in some cases with difficulties experienced in meeting partners during the lockdown.

In another US study, gay and bisexual men and other men who said they had sex with men were questioned about the sexual practices during the pandemic as compared with before it. Data were collected from over 500 men through an online survey conducted in February, March and April 2020 when the United States was largely locked down (Stephenson et al., 2021). Respondents were asked about their number of sexual partners, number of anal sex partners and number of unprotected sexual partners. Two-thirds of this sample believed it was possible to be infected with COVID-19 through sexual interaction. Most did not think it was essential to reduce their number of sexual partners during the pandemic, but recognised the need to be more cautious about their sexual behaviour. Anal sex, however, was rated as the least risky sex act.

On average, these men reported an increase in their number of sexual partners and of anal sexual partners during this period and hardly any change in the number of unprotected sexual partners. The increase in partners averaged two in a range of 40–70. Increased sexual activity was also associated with increased substance abuse and binge drinking during this period.

The sexual risks taken by men that sleep with other men are often linked to other risk factors, such as the use of illegal drugs. This relationship was confirmed by research conducted during the pandemic. Users of drugs such as cocaine/crack, methamphetamine, MDMA/ecstasy and ketamine were more inclined to engage in higher risk sexual behaviour, having more partners and taking fewer precautions.

A pre-pandemic baseline survey sample provides a point of comparison with a much smaller sample recruited during the pandemic. In general, sexual practices remained stable across pre-pandemic and pandemic for most original respondents. For the smaller COVID sample, however, sexual promiscuity and unprotected sexual practices among these men who had sex with other men were both likely to increase among those continuing to take hard drugs. Sexual risks did not exhibit any general increase during the pandemic, except for those men taking illegal drugs where risk practices did grow (Starks et al., 2020).

Another survey of men, in Israel, who had sex with other men showed that four in ten (40%) said they continued to meet casual sex partners during the early pandemic period in 2020 (Shilo & Mor, 2020). This behaviour was especially prevalent among young, single men and was linked to reporting higher levels of mental distress during social distancing and isolation restrictions. However, there were some signs of risk aversion with reports among some of the men that they had reduced some sexual practices, such as kissing. There was further evidence that some switched to other forms of sexual and social gratification by increasing their use of online dating sites, sex phone chats, webcams and pornography. Interestingly, during this early stage of the pandemic, these men did experience severe threat from COVID-19 with far fewer saying they could imagine having sex with someone infected (3%) compared to those saying this about someone with HIV (30%).

Turning to overt sexual behaviour, men and the gay community were more likely to report increased sexual activity than were women and heterosexual people. Single people and casual daters were more likely than those in established relationships to report decreases in sexual behaviour than were those in pre-lockdown established relationships. General health conditions and changes in subjective well-being, that is, how healthy and well people felt themselves to be, exhibited no statistically significant relationship to sexual desire or the propensity to sleep with others in a causal way (Wignall et al., 2021).

"Sociosexuality", that is, open sexual behaviour with different sexual partners, where it was still possible, made female, but not male participants, feel better in subjective health terms. In contrast, those individuals with a greater desire for casual sex reported more subjectively negative consequences of lockdown restrictions where it limited their usual sexual behaviour than did those who did not desire casual sex (see also, Jacob et al., 2020; Stephenson et al., 2020).

Given that sociosexuality is defined by individuals physically interacting at close quarters with strangers or people they do not live with, lockdown restrictions did target such activity among others via social isolation rules. It is likely therefore that people for whom casual sex is a regular part of their lives would feel the effects of being prohibited from engaging in such behaviour. If a targeted approach to controlling the spread of the coronavirus became core policy as the world emerged from lockdown, but with the virus still in circulation, devotees to sociosexuality would need to be among those targeted.

Some commentators on this matter have advised that public health authorities would need to be subtle in the COVID-related health education strategies they adopt with such people given already-existing prejudices against this behaviour among large factions of many populations (Vrangalova et al., 2015; Sanchez et al., 2020). Another reason for a cautious approach here is reinforced by evidence that among some sexually liberal communities COVID-related restrictions on close physical interactions could lead to the emergence of other harmful behaviours such as excessive alcohol consumption (Stephenson et al., 2020).

Lockdown and Relationship Strain

Many people reported at least some degree of psychological distress caused by the pandemic. In some instances, this response could be severe. It was shaped not just by concern about the risks of infection and the seriousness of illness that might follow, but also by the constraints imposed on their everyday behaviour by the lockdown. Hence, many populations suffered widespread pandemic-related and lockdown-related stress. This experience was unpleasant for the individual and could also affect others around them. People living together who were forced to spend much more time in the same physical space than they would normally could experience stress within their close personal relationships. While some couples might have found lockdown a bonding experience, especially if they had not previously spent a lot of time together, for others it could give rise to tensions boiling over sometimes into conflict. Hence, some partners learned to appreciate each other more and others came to loath one another. Such reactions raise questions about the overall impact of the pandemic on relationships.

One American analysis by the Institute for Family Studies of divorce filings in five states between January and August 2020 inclusive reported decreased filings at the peak of the pandemic (in March to April 2020). Over later months, as many parts of the country emerged from lockdown, there was evidence that divorce filings rates increased again (Seidman, 2020). A different picture emerged from another investigation that found no strong evidence of relationship declines as state lockdowns were put in place. This research detected a lesser tendency in lockdown for one partner to criticise the other for intentionally engaging in what they saw as "bad behaviour". The lockdown seemed to have generated a psychological climate in which one partner was more understanding of the moods of the other and recognised that they were both dealing with a difficult situation for which neither was ultimately to blame. Hence, there was greater tolerance and forgiveness in the air. In general, couples that experienced the most severe strains on their relationships during the pandemic were those who were not getting on so well before it (Williamson, 2020).

In spite of this reassuring finding, the same research revealed that relationship satisfaction did not invariably remain stable. For some couples, it improved and for others, it got worse. The key triggers were income level, whether a couple was married or not and whether their experience of the pandemic was, on balance, negative or positive in terms of their income level and their dislike of social isolation from others. What was then critical was whether a couple worked out a way of being mutually supportive through these trying times. This supportiveness was also linked back to how one partner attributed causes to the others problematic pandemic responses. There were indications that couples that ended up in open conflict generally exhibited poorer initial relationship satisfaction levels were probably experiencing relationship problems before the pandemic (Williamson, 2020).

In summing up, therefore, the pandemic could have both positive and negative effects on people's personal relationships. These responses depended upon the stability of their lives and their relationship at the outset of the pandemic and their government's introduction of behaviour restrictions. As the next chapter will show sometimes these relationship tensions can boil over into highly toxic and destructive behaviour patterns with very serious consequences for all those involved.

References

Aarts, S., Peek, S. T. M., & Wouters, E. J. M. (2015). The relation between social network site usage and loneliness and mental health in community-dwelling older adults. *International Journal of Geriatric Psychiatry*, 30(9): 942–949.

Balzarini, R., Muise, A., Zoppolat, G., Bartolomeo, A., Rodrigues, D., Alonso-Ferres, M., Urganci, B., Debrot, A., Pichayayothin, N., Dharma, C., Chi, P., Karremans, J., Schoebi, D., & Slatcher, R. (2020). *Love in the time of COVID: Perceived partner responsiveness buffers people from lower relationship quality associated with COVID-related stressors.* PsyArXiv. doi: 10.31234/osf.io/e3fh4

Beaver, K., Pedley, K., & Garrett, C. (2020, 18th November). Young Britons most likely to break Coronanvirus rules in pursuit of romance. Ipsos-MORI. Retrieved from: https://www.ipsos.com/ipsos-mori/en-uk/young-britons-most-likely-break-coronavirus-rules-pursuit-romance-0

BPS (2020, 30th November). *Covid-19 and Intimate Relationships*. The British Psychological Society. Retrieved from: https://www.bps.org.uk/sites/www.bps.org.uk/files/Policy/Policy%20-%20Files/Covid-19%20and%20intimate%20relationships.pdf

Butterworth, B. (2021, 16th April). Dating after lockdown: How the COVID rules on romance are easing – and when people can have sex. *I News*. Retrieved from: https://inews.co.uk/news/uk/dating-lockdown-covid-rules-easing-when-have-sex-again-960179

Cito G., Micelli E., Cocci A., Polloni G., Russo G. I., Coccia M. E., Simoncini T., Carini M., Minervini A., & Natali A. (2021). The impact of the COVID-19 quarantine on sexual life in Italy. *Urology*. 147: 37–42. doi: 10.1016/j.urology.2020.06.101

Collins, C., Landivar, L. C., Ruppanner, L., & Scarborough, W. J. (2021). COVID-19 and the gender gap in work hours. *Gender, Work, and Organization*, 28(S1): 101–112. doi: 10.1111/gwao.12506

Coombe J., Kong F. Y. S., Bittleston H., Williams H., Tomnay J., Vaisey A., Malta S., Goller J. L., Temple-Smith M., Bourchier L., Lau A., Chow E. P. F., & Hocking J. S. (2020). Love during lockdown: findings from an online survey examining the impact of COVID-19 on the sexual health of people living in Australia. *Sexually Transmitted Infections*, sextrans-2020-054688. doi: 10.1136/sextrans-2020-054688

Duncan, S., Phillips, M., Roseneil, S., Carter, J., & Stoilova, M. (2013). *Living apart together: Uncoupling intimacy and co-residence* [Research Briefing]. NatCen Social Research. https://natcen.ac.uk/media/28546/living-apart-together.pdf

Fang, D., Peng, J., Liao, S., Tang, Y., Cui, W., Yuan, Y., Wiu, D., Hu, B., Wang, R., Song, W., Gao, B., Jin, L., & Zhang, Z. (2021). An online questionnaire survey on the sexual life and sexual function of Chinese adult men during the coronavirus disease 2019 epidemic. *Sexual Medicine*, 9(1): 100293.

French, J. E., Altgelt, E. E., & Meltzer, A. L. (2019). The implications of socio-sexuality for marital satisfaction and dissolution. *Psychological Science*, 30(10): 1460–1472. doi: 10.1177/0956797619868997

Gausman, J., & Langer, A. (2020). Sex and gender disparities in the COVID-19 pandemic. *Journal of Women's Health*, 29(4): 465–466. doi: 10.1089/jwh.2020.8472

GDI (2020, 18th May). Research shows UK daters are more polite and creative during lockdown. https://www.globaldatinginsights.com/news/research-shows-uk-daters-are-more-polite-and-creative-during-lockdown

Hawkley, L. C., Burleson, M. H., Berntson, G. G., & Cacioppo, J. T. (2003). Loneliness in everyday life: Cardiovascular activity, psychosocial context, and health behaviours. *Journal of Personality and Social Psychology*, 85(1): 105–120. doi: 10.1037/0022-3514.85.1.105

Ibarra, F. P., Mehrad, M., Di Mauro, M., Godoy, M. F. P., Cruz, E. G., Nilforoushzadeh, M. A., & Russo, G. I. (2020). Impact of the COVID-19 pandemic on the sexual behaviour of the population. The vision of the east and the west. *International Brazilian Journal of Urology*, 46(suppl. 1): 104–112.

Jacob, L., Smith, L., Butler, L., Barnett, Y., Grabovac, I., McDermott, D., Armstrong, N., Yakkundi, A., & Tully, M. (2020). Challenges in the practice of sexual medicine in the time of COVID-19 in the United Kingdom. *Journal of Sexual Medicine*, 17(7): 1229–1236. doi: 10.1016/j.jsxm.2020.05.001

Jowett, A. (2020). The psychological impact of social distancing on gender, sexuality and relationship diverse populations. *Psychology of Sexualities Section Review*, 11(1): 6–8.

Lehmiller, J., Garcia, J., Gesselman, A., & Mark, K. (2021). Less sex, but more sexual diversity: Changes in sexual behaviour during the COVID-19 coronavirus pandemic. *Leisure Sciences*, 43(1–2), 295–304. https://doi.org/10.1080/01490400.2020.1774016

Lenzer, J. (2020). Covid-19: US gives emergency approval to hydroxychloroquine despite lack of evidence. *BMJ*, 369: m1335. doi: 10.1136/bmj.m1335

Levin, I. (2004). Living apart together: A new family form. *Current Sociology*, 52(2): 223–240. doi: 10.1177/0011392104041809

Li W., Li G., Xin C., Wang Y., & Yang S. (2020). Challenges in the Practice of Sexual Medicine in the Time of COVID-19 in China. *Journal of Sexual Medicine*, 17(7): 1225–1228. doi: 10.1016/j.jsxm.2020.04.380

Li, L. Z., & Wang, S. (2020). Prevalence and predictors of general psychiatric disorders and loneliness during COVID-19 in the United Kingdom. *Psychiatry Research*, 291: 11 3267. doi: 10.1016/j.psychres.2020.113267

Li, W., Li, G., Xin, C., Wang, Y., & Yang, S. (2020). Challenges in the practice of sexual medicine in the time of COVID-19 in China. *Journal of Sexual Medicine*, 17(7): 1225–1228. doi: 10.1016/j.jsxm.2020.04.380

Lopes de Sousa, A. F., Braz de Oliveira Nune Queiroz, A. A. F. L., Felix de Csevalho, H. E., Schneider, G., Cmargo, E. L. S., Evangelista de Aruajo, T. M., Brignol, S., Mendes, I. A. C., Fronteira, I., & McFarland, W. (2021). Casual sex among men who have sex with men (MSM) during the period of sheltering in place to prevent the spread of COVID-19. *International Journal of Environmental Research and Public Health*, 18(6): 3266. doi: 10.3390/ijerph18063266

López-Bueno, R., López Sánchez, G. F., Gil-Salmeron, A., Grabovac, I., Tully, M. A., Casana, J., & Smith, L. (2021). COVID-19 confinement and sexual activity in Spain: A cross-sectional study. *International Journal of Environmental Research and Public Health*, 18(5): 2559. doi: 10.3390/ijerph18052559

Matthews, T., Danese, A., Gregory, A. M., Caspi, A., Moffitt, T. E., & Arseneault, L. (2017). Sleeping with one eye open: Loneliness and sleep quality in young adults. *Psychological Medicine*, 47(12): 2177–2186. doi: 10.1017/S0033291717000629

Mitchell, K., Shimonovich, M., Boso Perez, R., Clifton, S., Tanton, C., Macdowell, W., Bonell, C., Riddell, J., Copas, A., Sonnenberg, P., Marcer, C., & Field, N. (2020). Early impacts of COVID-19 on sex life and relationship quality: Findings from a large British quasi-representative online survey (Natsal-COVID). *BMJ*, 97(1). doi: 10.1136/sextrans-2021-sti.76

Nolsoe, E. (2020, 12th June). Sex and dating under COVID-19. *YouGov*. Retrieved from: https://yougov.co.uk/topics/relationships/articles-reports/2020/06/12/sex-and-dating-under-covid-19

Overall, N., Chang, V., Pietromonaco, P., Low, R., & Henderson, A. (2020). *Relationship functioning during COVID-19 quarantine*. PsyArXiv. doi: 10.31234/osf.io/7cvdm

Pebody, R. (2021, 22nd April). What happened to people's sex lives during lockdown in Britain? *nam aidsmap*. Retrieved from: https://www.aidsmap.com/news/apr-2021/what-happened-peoples-sex-lives-during-lockdown-britain

Pietromonaco, P. R., & Beck, L. A. (2019). Adult attachment and physical health. *Current Opinion in Psychology*, 25: 115–120. doi: 10.1016/j.copsyc.2018.04.004

Pietromonaco, P., & Collins, N. L. (2017). Interpersonal mechanisms linking close relationships to health. *American Psychologist*, 72(6): 531–5424. doi: 10.1037/amp0000129

Public Health England. (2020). *Coronavirus (COVID 19)*. Gov.uk. Retrieved August 13th, 2020, from https://publichealthmatters.blog.gov.uk/category/coronavirus-covid-19/

Raque-Bogdan, T. L., Ericson, S. K., Jackson, J., Martin, H. M., & Bryan, N. A. (2011). Attachment and mental and physical health: Self-compassion and mattering as mediators. *Journal of Counseling Psychology*, 58(2): 272–278. doi: 10.1037/a0023041

Rodrigues, D., Lopes, D., & Smith, C. V. (2017). Caught in a "Bad Romance"? Reconsidering the negative association between sociosexuality and relationship functioning. *Journal of Sex Research*, 54(9): 1118–1127. doi: 10.1080/00224499.2016.1252308

Sánchez, O. R., Vale, D. B., Rodrigues, L., & Surita, F. G. (2020). Violence against women during the COVID-19 pandemic: An integrative review. *International Journal of Gynecology & Obstetrics*, 151(2): 180–187. doi: https://doi.org/10.1002/ijgo.13365

Seidman, G. (2020, 18th December). Has COVID-19 helped or harmed romantic relationships? *Psychology Today*. Retrieved from: https://www.psychologytoday.com/us/blog/close-encounters/202012/has-covid-19-helped-or-harmed-romantic-relationships

Shaw, D. (2020, 21st May). *Coronavirus: Tinder Boss Says Dramatic Changes to Dating*. BBC News. Retrieved from: https://www.bbc.co.uk/news/business-52743454

Schiavi, M. C., Spina, V., Zullo, M. A., Colagiovanni, V., Luffarelli, P., Rago, R., & Palazzetti, P. (2020). Love in the time of COVID-19: Sexual function and quality of life analysis during the social distancing measures in a group of Italian reproductive-age women. *Journal of Sexual Medicine*, 17(8): 1407–1413.

Shilo, G., & Mor, Z. (2020). COVID-19 and the changes in the sexual behavior of men who have sex with men: Results of an online survey. *Journal of Sexual Medicine*, 17(10): 1827–1834. https://doi.org/10.1016/j.jsxm.2020.07.085

Simpson, J. A., & Gangestad, S. W. (1991). Individual differences in sociosexuality: Evidence for convergent and discriminant validity. *Journal of Personality and Social Psychology*, 60(6): 870–883. doi: 10.1037/0022-3514.60.6.870

Starks, T. J., Jones, S. S., Sauermilch, D., Benedict, M., Adebayo, T., Cain, D., & Simpson, K. N. (2020). Evaluating the impact of COVID-19: A cohort comparison study of drug use and risk sexual behavior among sexual minority men in the U. S. A. *Drug and Alcohol Dependency*, 216: 108260. doi: 10.1016/j.drugalcdep.2020.108260.

Stephenson, R., Chavanduka, T. M., Rosso, M. T., Sullivan, S. P., Pitter, R. A., Hunter, A. S., & Rogers, E. (2020). Sex in the time of COVID-19: Results of an online survey of gay, bisexual and other men who have sex with men's experience of sex and HIV prevention during the US COVID-19 epidemic. *AIDS and Behavior*, 25(1): 40–48. doi: 10.1007/s10461-020-03024-8

Stephenson, T., Shafran, R., De Stavola, B., Rojas, N., Aiano, F., Amin-Chowdhury, Z., McOwat, K., Simmons, R., Zavala, M., Consortium, C., & Ladhani, S. N. (2021). Long COVID and the mental and physical health of children and young people: national matched cohort study protocol (the CLoCk study). *BMJ Open*, 11(8): e052838. doi: 10.1136/bmjopen-2021-052838

Ugurlucan, F. G., Yasa, C., Tikiz, M. A., Evruke, I., Isik, C., Durai, O., & Akhan, S. E. (2021). Effect of the COVID-19 pandemic and social distancing measures on the sexual functions of women treated for vaginismus (genitopelvic pain/penetration disorder). *International Urogynecology Journal*, 1–7. doi: 10.1007/s00192-020-04667-w

Usher, K., Bhullar, N., Durkin, J., Gyamfi, N., & Jackson, D. (2020). Family violence and COVID-19: Increased vulnerability and reduced options for support. *International Journal of Mental Health Nursing*, 29(4): 549–552. doi: 10.1111/inm.12735

Van Bilsen, W. P. H., Zimmermann, H. M. L., Boyd, A., Coyer, L., van der Hoek, L., Koostra, N. A., Hoonenborg, E., Prins, M., van der Loeff, M. F. S., Davidovich, U., & Matser. A. (2021). Sexual behaviour and its determinants during COVID-19 restrictions among men who have sex with men in Amsterdam. *Journal of Acquired Immune Deficiency Syndrome*, 86(3): 288–296.

Vrangalova, Z., Bukberg, R. E., & Rieger, G. (2015). Birds of a feather? Not when it comes to sexual permissiveness. *Journal of Social and Personal Relationships*, 31(1): 93–113. doi: 10.1177/0265407513487638.

Vrangalova, Z., & Ong, A. D. (2014). Who benefits from casual sex? The moderating role of sociosexuality. *Social Psychological and Personality Science*, 5(8): 883–891. doi: 10.1177/1948550614537308

Walsh, A. R., Sullivan, S., & Stephenson, R. (2021). Are male couples changing their sexual agreements and behaviors during the COVID-19 pandemic? *AIDS Behaviour*, 1–6. doi: 10.1007/s10461-021-03256-2

Wignall, L., & McCormack, M. (2021, 30th March). How lockdown changed the sex lives of young adults – new research. *The Conversation*. https://www. theconversation.com/how-lockdown-changed-the-sex-lives-of-young-adults-new-research-156873

Wignall, L., Portch, E. McComrack, M., Owens, R., Cascalheira, C. J., & Attard-Johnson, J. (2021). Changes in sexual desire and behaviours among young adults during social lockdown dues to COVID-19. *Journal of Sex Research*, doi: 10.1080/00224499.2021.1897067

Williamson, H. C. (2020). Early effects of COVID-19 pandemic in relationship satisfaction and attributions. *Psychological Science*, 31(12). doi: 10.1177/095 6797620972688

Chapter 8

The Pandemic and Destructive Behaviour

Social distancing rules during the pandemic meant that people were starved of social and physical contact. Among the concerns were how the frustrations caused by these restrictions could boil over into anger and aggression. Many potentially harmful behaviours could flow from this. Sometimes, these behaviours were targeted at others and sometimes inwardly by people towards themselves. Much aggression triggered by the pandemic was likely to be projected onto other people living under the same roof. This possibility meant that already concerning levels of domestic abuse might increase. There was then an additional concern about anxiety, depression and frustration being turned inwards towards self-harm. Evidence started to emerge that for some already troubled individuals, this state of affairs could trigger extreme behavioural responses including suicide (Courtet et al., 2020). This chapter will examine both of these behaviour side-effects.

Self-Harm

Being isolated from others meant that many people lost their social support systems through which they received emotional sustenance and also obtained information from trusted sources that would enable them cognitively to develop coping mechanisms to reduce the uncertainties around COVID-19. Writing early on in the pandemic, Courtet and his colleagues advised that care systems needed as a matter of urgency to find ways of helping isolated people to cope better with the pandemic by devising distractions as well as by offering reassurance (Courtet et al., 2020).

The concerns about more extreme and potentially harmful reactions to the pandemic and lockdown interventions were especially acute in regard to older people. Many older people might already have been isolated from others, short of friends and marginalised by families. The restrictions of lockdown required them to keep their social distance from others and, if infected or in close contact with others who were infected, to quarantine and effectively be placed under house arrest with no social contact at all. Any mental health side-effects could then become very severe and for those

DOI: 10.4324/9781003274377-8

elderly who were frightened by what was happening to an extreme degree, there could be longer-term behaviour-debilitating effects (Holt et al., 2020; Wand et al., 2020).

Among the critical side-effects of the pandemic were the postponement of essential treatments for patients with a range of illnesses and health conditions as health professionals and facilities were directed exclusively or mostly to dealing with COVID-19. For patients in severe pain or suffering from life-threatening conditions, the anxiety and frustration caused by the absence of much-needed treatment could drive some to despair and then to seek more extreme solutions to end their discomfort (Wand et al., 2018). At the same time, these individuals might also feel they have become a burden on their families, carers and society during a time when everyone is suffering from the effects of a major global health crisis. Such feelings can further disrupt their own mental state and create a mindset that leads them to self-harm (Wand et al., 2018; Wand & Perisah, 2020). Reports also emerged during the pandemic that in addition to an upsurge in self-harm behaviour there were also increased requests for voluntary assisted dying (Lapid et al., 2020).

Suicidal Behaviour

Before reviewing the findings of pandemic studies of suicide behaviour, it is important to set out the different classes of suicidal response ranging from thought processes to actual harmful behaviour. Sometimes people have thoughts about injuring themselves when they are feeling down but they never act upon them. Such thoughts might graduate to those specifically about ending one's life (suicide ideation). Moving from just thinking about self-harm, some individuals might engage in mild self-harming behaviours that are not life-threatening but do attract attention. At the furthest extreme in the direction of increased harm, there are a few people that might actually try to end their lives. These might be unsuccessful (attempted suicide) or successful (suicide) (Nock et al., 2008; Ghazinour et al., 2010; Sveticic & De Leo, 2012).

One theory (Interpersonal Theory of Suicide) has posited that thinking about suicide can lead to attempted suicide (Joiner, 2005). Another theory (Integrated Motivational-Volitional Model) has proposed that the process from thought to life-ending behaviour is not as simple and direct as that. Instead, there may be several stages whereby suicidal thoughts might lead to self-harming that is not initially life-threatening and may never develop further, but then sometimes it can (O'Connor, 2011).

While having thoughts about suicide might seem to many people to be so problematic that it surely cannot be very prevalent, research into the topic has indicated that around the world as many as one in seven (14%) of people reported having such thoughts (Biswas et al., 2020) and twice this proportion (30%) has been found among young adults (Evans et al., 2005). When it comes to non-life-threatening self-injurious behaviour, the prevalence was found to vary from 6% to 17% in the lifetime of people living in different parts of the world (Swannell et al., 2014).

Suicide is a serious matter at any time. Evidence emerged during the pandemic in the United Kingdom that it had had an adverse effect on the mental health of lots of people. Surveys recorded reports of deterioration in a variety of psychological conditions known to play a part in facilitating suicidal thoughts (Fancourt et al., 2020; O'Connor et al., 2020; Pierce et al., 2020). Risk factors included increased isolation and loneliness, removal of normal mental health care support, bereavement, domestic violence, alcohol abuse and economic hardship (Gunnell et al., 2020).

Suicide rates had been found to increase in previous pandemics. Research in Hong Kong at the time of the SARS (Severe Acute Respiratory Syndrome) coronavirus outbreak in 2003 showed that the suicide rate among people aged 65 and over increased during the pandemic compared with the year before and also compared with an earlier period spanning the mid-1980s to mid-1990s. The increased suicide rate among this age group was mostly accounted for by women (Chan et al., 2006).

The pressures many people felt during the COVID-19 pandemic, however, led to the numbers contemplating ending their lives growing by worrying margins in a number of countries such as Japan, Nepal, Norway and Peru (Calderon-Anyosa & Kaufman, 2021; Pokhrel & Chhetri 2021; Qin & Mehlum, 2020; Ueda et al., 2020). Elsewhere in Australia, England and Massachusetts, United States suicide rates remained largely unchanged during the pandemic (Coroners Court of Victoria, 2020; Appleby et al., 2021; Faust et al., 2021).

One study carried out in England in 2020 found no evidence of increased suicide rates during the early phase of the pandemic. An average of 121.3 suicides per month were recorded from April to October 2020 after the first lockdown began. This compared with 125.7 per month from January to March 2020 before that lockdown had fully got underway. Suicide rates did not suddenly increase during April and May 2020 when the first lockdown was in place and this situation did not change over the next five months as the United Kingdom came out of lockdown. Further comparisons between 2020 data and suicide rates recorded in 2019 showed no significant change (Appleby et al., 2021).

A longitudinal study in Ireland in May 2020 and then again in August 2020 found nearly three in ten (30%) said they had entertained suicidal thoughts (known as "suicidal ideation") at some point in their lives, a further one in seven (13%) had engaged in suicidal self-injury and just over one in ten (11%) had attempted suicide. These figures may seem high but were in fact in line with reports of these behaviours in other parts of the world (Evans et al., 2005; Swannell et al., 2014).

The result just reported also mirrored findings of a study of more than 3,000 British adults conducted between March to May 2020 (O'Connor et al., 2020). There was evidence of an increase in rates of having suicidal thoughts over the period of the study most especially among young people. The proportion of young people saying they had had these thoughts during the early phase of the pandemic (14%) was slightly up on pre-pandemic levels for this age group (11%) (O'Connor et al., 2018). No evidence emerged, however, that self-injury rates changed during the pandemic, but where it did occur, it was more likely among males, the unemployed, those with reportedly higher levels of loneliness and individuals who were not very religious. Non-suicidal self-injury was linked to a history of mental health problems. Attempted suicide was more prevalent among ethnic minorities, individuals with lower levels of education and lower income, sufferers from post-traumatic stress and those with depression.

Further analysis showed that among at least two-thirds of those who reported suicide ideation, there was no subsequent conversion of these thoughts into non-suicidal injurious tendencies or attempted suicide. Furthermore, virtually all of those individuals who said they had engaged in non-suicidal personal injury (96%) or attempted suicide (97%) had not previously entertained thoughts about suicide. This does not mean that suicide ideation is never related to attempted suicide because there was pre-pandemic research evidence to show that it could be (Neeleman et al., 2004; Klonsky et al., 2016; Ribeiro et al., 2016; Mars et al., 2019), early inter-vention with these cases can help to reduce the likelihood of harmful thoughts being translated into harmful behaviour (Tarrier et al., 2008; Geddes et al., 2013). It should also be noted that these pandemic studies covered relatively limited periods of time and do not provide clear evidence of the longer-term effects of suicidal ideation. Being mindful that people who are hospitalised because of their suicidal thoughts are likely to keep having these thoughts unless appropriate steps are taken, psychotherapeutically, to mitigate against them (Windsor et al., 2015; Bryant et al., 2017).

Domestic Abuse

One of the biggest concerns in terms of behavioural side-effects of the pandemic was the rise in domestic violence. With lockdown and other re-strictions requiring people to stay home more and with workplace and school closures resulting in adults and children being home together more of the time, a recipe was struck for arguments and tensions to occur especially when space was restricted. Research in the United States found that one in five parents (20%) admitted to having hit their child in the previous two weeks after the coronavirus had been declared a pandemic. Parents that reacted badly to social isolation and whose jobs had been lost or were under threat were more inclined to show their frustrations in this way. The more time parents spent in lockdown situations, the more likely they were to vent their pent-up tensions in the form of overt aggression.

For every extra day spent under social distancing restrictions, there was a 14% increase in the likelihood that a parent had smacked their child in the previous two weeks. These effects were still present after parents pre-existing depressive symptoms or disciplinary practices were controlled (Lee & Ward, 2020; Lee et al., 2020). Mothers specifically were found to be more likely to hit their children to control their behaviour across the course of pandemic-related restrictions on their normal lives (Rodriguez et al., 2020).

The stresses caused also by the need for parents or carers to get involved in home schooling their children while also doing their own work from home created further complications for many families. Adults in the home might also be under pressure because they feel their own jobs are at risk as many employers folded their businesses as their revenues crashed because their customers were not able to go out and use their services or simply stopped spending money because of uncertainties over their own future employment. The absence of stress releasors found in entertainment and leisure activities and in simply being allowed to mix socially with other people also created greater intra-family strains which could become manifest in internalised anxiety or externalised aggression (Lee, 2020).

The stress caused by lockdown restrictions, underpinned by people worrying about family members getting ill as well as being fearful of this for themselves, and then the many spin-off side-effects such as loss of income, loss of job, loss of social contact and loss of normal daily routines, could, for some people, become debilitating. For others, the frustrations that resulted boiled over into other behaviour patterns that were altogether more disruptive and could pose real risks to others. One specific area of concern, that arose from spikes in normally troublesome conduct, was domestic violence (Humphreys et al., 2020).

When those sharing a home were forced to spend more time together than they would do under more usual circumstances, opportunities were increased for COVID-related tensions to spill over into increased antagonism between them. Partners that already had a track record of domestic abuse might be more likely to behave this way. The increased presence of children in the home during daytime hours because of school closures meant that they too might find themselves in the firing line of these violent outbursts. There was much pre-COVID evidence that child abuse often intersected with other domestic abuse such as between spouses and partners. This violence was increasingly likely to occur among specific personality types, but could also be aggravated by local circumstances (Herrenkohl et al., 2008; Wildeman et al., 2014; Vu et al., 2016). Being socially isolated or quarantined was known to increase anger levels especially among those individuals with stronger internal dispositions to behave aggressively. Draconian restrictions on people's behaviour and constantly changing rules concerning restrictions could cause confusion and stressful uncertainty (Brooks et al., 2020).

The research found that dramatic changes to normal routines could be upsetting to young children and difficult for them to cope with. This might then lead to them displaying attention-seeking behaviour that triggers severe responses from parents. If parents are already in a state of high-stress arousal, there could be outbursts of temper that can lead to verbal and physical abuse (Humphreys et al., 2020).

The problem of domestic abuse was already established worldwide and the global pandemic resulted in reports of widespread increases in this behaviour. The ubiquitous deployment of preventive measures such as encouraging people to stay home and to keep their social distance from others from outside their home created conditions under which adverse mental reactions were commonplace and principally experienced within the home. One study from Ethiopia reported one in four women of child-bearing age (25%) experienced violence from an intimate partner. In around half of these cases, the "violence" was psychological and in one in five cases it was sexual. In nearly one-third of cases, it was physical. This behaviour was most prevalent among women aged under-30 and in arranged marriages (Gebrewahd et al., 2020).

Lockdown and Domestic Abuse

As couples were forced to spend more time together at home than usual during the pandemic, tension could build in relationships that in turn could boil over in conflict and violence. Research in Greater London during COVID-19 lockdown detected some shifts in patterns of domestic abuse during this time, but, to some degree, this shift also reflected changes in the way this behaviour was reported. In general, there were increases found in abuse perpetrated by current partners and family members (by margins of 8% and 17% respectively), abuse by former partners declined (–11%). The latter behaviour, of course, was probably affected by restrictions on public behaviour and especially on meetings between people from different households. In contrast, the pressures caused by lockdown in many family households catalysed abusive behaviour between people living together, often because they spent more time than usual in each other's company. In terms of cases coming to the attention of the authorities, this study found that during lockdown there was probably some degree of underreporting of these incidents. Once again, the reduction in social contact between households meant there were fewer opportunities for outsiders – who may have reported abuse – to become aware of it (Ivandic & Kirchmaier, 2020; Ivandic et al., 2020).

Ivandic and Kirchmaier analysed five years of criminal records and two years of calls-for-service data from the London Metropolitan Police Service (MPS) up to 14th June 2020. The MPS received an average of 2.5 million calls a year and of these around seven per cent were related to domestic abuse. The researchers found that since the beginning of the first United Kingdom-wide lockdown which began on the 23rd March 2020 to the 14th June 2020, the MPS received around 45,000 domestic abuse calls. Compared to the same period in 2019, this represented a significant year-on-year increase in calls to the police of over 11%. Much of this increase, however, comprised calls from third parties who had not directly witnessed incidents, but had nonetheless become aware of them. In these instances, the indirect witnesses might have heard noises from their neighbours or seen some of the consequences to victims.

There was further evidence that not all types of domestic abuse increased during the lockdown and some even dropped. In London, the Metropolitan police reported more third-party calls reporting domestic incidents during the first lockdown period and explained this as being a function of more people spending time at home in adjacent premises where these incidents could be overheard. There was also an increase in demand for domestic abuse support services at this time, providing further evidence of a surge in activity. This did not necessarily mean there were more incidents, but possibly that there were greater numbers of serious incidents leading victims to seek outside help. Social distancing measures would also have curtailed opportunities for support from family members living elsewhere and from friends.

During the three years leading up to the pandemic, domestic abuse offences per month across England and Wales were found to have increased. As well as changes in police reporting measures, there may also have been a greater willingness on the part of victims to come forward and report abuse. From March to June 2020, the police recorded 259,324 offences classed as domestic abuse. This was an increase of 7% in the same period in 2019 and an 18% increased on the same months in 2018. Given that the 2020 figures represented a continuation of an upward trend already occurring pre-pandemic, it cannot be concluded from these data alone that domestic abuse cases increased during the pandemic possibly because of the collateral psychological damage of lockdown.

Monthly data for April (21%), May (20%) and June (19%) showed the proportion of all offences recorded by the police that were classed as domestic abuse. The proportions of domestic offences subsequently began to decline as lockdown restrictions were released over the summer months of 2020. However, this may have occurred because there had been a decrease in all recorded crime during the lockdown and this started to move again once restrictions were relaxed. When domestic abuse cases were represented as a proportion of all violence against the person offences between March and June 2020, a 9% increase was recorded compared with the same period in 2019 (Office of National Statistics, 2020).

Other evidence emerged internationally that cases of violence between intimate partners did exhibit increased prevalence during the pandemic (Giussy et al., 2020). The pressures of the pandemic's restrictions on behaviour might aggravate the aggressive predispositions of the violent partner. At the same time, the victim (often not always female) could not easily escape the abusive environment because of the same restrictions. Any apparent decrease or stability in domestic abuse cases might also be explained in terms of the propensity of victims to report these incidents. Evidence emerged from Italy, for example, that women had been less willing to come forward to report these incidents during the pandemic (Giussy et al., 2020).

Reports also emerged of intimate partner violence in remote regions of northern Canada. This behaviour was not unknown there, but the restrictions introduced by the Canadian government to bring the spread of COVID-19 under control made matters worse. Domestic violence cases were already worse in these regions than in large cities (Moffitt et al., 2020).

Mental Health and Domestic Abuse

Domestic abuse does not occur in a psychological vacuum. It is behaviour that is often linked to wider mental health problems among people that live together. Some mental health problems can exacerbate the frustrations caused by high-stress settings or lead to destructive rather than constructive coping responses (Oram et al., 2013a, 2013b).

Pre-pandemic evidence had indicated that psychiatric problems were prevalent in domestic abuse cases and especially ones that resulted in homicides. Data for the England and Wales had shown that nearly one in four (23%) of perpetrators of domestic homicides had been in touch with mental health services during the year before the offence and one in three perpetrators (34%) were found that have psychiatric problems at the time of their offence (Oram et al., 2013b). These links between serious domestic abuse incidents and mental health problems were corroborated beyond the United Kingdom (Yu et al., 2020).

Delving deeper into the research, however, revealed that even though there were frequent associations between occurrences of mental health problems and domestic abuse cases, there was no compelling evidence that specific mental states were the primary causes of this violent behaviour. Often there were other factors in play such as substance abuse and other family dynamics, sometimes linked to cultural values and family relationship conventions (Bhavsar et al., 2021).

Once again, observations were made by experts in the field that mental health services were confronted with a really serious challenge in monitoring domestic abuse because during lockdown the opportunities for such cases to gain external visibility had been curtailed. Health services were directed towards combating the pandemic and many had been temporarily halted because of physical distancing restrictions. During this period, therefore, mental health support was much reduced across the board and not just in relation to interventions in domestic abuse cases (Hester et al., 2019; Van Gelder et al., 2020). Enforced quarantines for extended periods in respect of those infected or suspected of being infected and the use of social isolation among those not yet infected, can disrupt normal life with damaging consequences which can become more pronounced the longer such restrictions are kept in place (Van Gelder et al., 2020).

These interventions also resulted in the withdrawal of professional support systems and family support networks. The stress caused by a pandemic and extreme measures to combat it, cause unpleasant mood states and if these conditions persist, more profound psychological effects are likely to be experienced (Zapor et al., 2015). The health consequences of these dynamics can be further aggravated by the absence of important social and emotional support networks (Brooks et al., 2020).

Loss of employment – for many temporarily and for some permanently – represented another significant stressor with its own psychological repercussions. Negative emotional responses to these circumstances can include anger or depression. Pent-up frustration needs to be vented somewhere and, in some households, this might occur in the form of violence of one member against another (Peterman et al., 2020).

Women as Victims

Domestic violence against women was flagged by the World Health Organization as one of the most serious collateral effects of the pandemic (WHO, 2020). Evidence accumulated from around the world of increased rates of domestic violence against women, with substantial increases being registered in China (+300%), Brazil (+50%), Cyprus, France and New Zealand (+25% each), the United Kingdom (+25%) and Spain (+20%) (Bradbury-Jones & Isham, 2020; Graham-Harrison et al., 2020; New Zealand Family Violence Clearinghouse, 2020). The incidence of violence against women in domestic settings could have been even higher in other countries, but there was a lack of reliable data to confirm this suspicion.

Violence against women can cause both physical and psychological harm that includes sexually transmitted diseases and unplanned pregnancies and, in the extreme, death (WHO, 2020). Most countries deployed preventive measures with COVID-19 that involved some degree of social isolation with people being required to stay home most of the time. With workplaces closed down, many people lost their jobs and their incomes which put households under considerable strain, with the frustration generated being released through violent outbursts frequently targeted at another household member (Norman et al., 2021; Tronick et al., 2021).

Reviews of research studies revealed a considerable body of evidence for the increased risks of violence against women in the home during the pandemic. Stay at home policies were described by some writers as creating a "pandemic within a pandemic". The other pandemic took the form of increased occurrences of violence against women often perpetrated by their partners at home (Viero et al., 2021).

In the United States, there was special concern about domestic abuse as a collateral side-effect of the pandemic restrictions among veterans, that is, former members of the armed forces. The risks of abusive relationships were known to be higher than average in households with veterans. Women veterans were especially at risk. The command to "stay home" for individuals accustomed to be away from home for extended periods, could place close relationships under great strain where the partners were unaccustomed to living together to that extent (Rossi et al., 2020).

Reporting on data from Europe and North America, researchers proposed that the extended and strict home confinement requirements of pandemic interventions in many high-income countries had created more dangerous domestic situations for some women. In some countries, this concern was borne out by data showing increased rates of this type of offence. There was an additional worry that this pattern might be repeated in less developed countries where domestic violence had historically been prevalent but where governments had not yet introduced severe societal lockdowns because infection levels did not yet warrant such interventions. Once this situation changed, however, women in abusive relationships could find themselves at greater physical risk (Tochie et al., 2020).

Men are also Abused

Two out of every three domestic abuse cases in the United Kingdom involved female victims (Office for National Statistics, 2019). This means that one in three involve male victims – a surprisingly high figure given that much popular attention is focused on female victims. Indeed, there is evidence to suggest that even this figure for men could be underestimation given the reluctance of male victims to come forward. Men (51%) were found to be much less likely to confide in some about their abuse than were women victims (81%) (Office of National Statistics, 2018). Men may feel embarrassed or ashamed about becoming victims of domestic abuse (Tsui et al., 2010).

The lockdowns deployed in the United Kindom during 2020–2021 pandemic confined many people to their own homes for much of the time. Many were encouraged to work from home or required by their employers to do so. Many others were laid off temporarily or permanently as businesses were required to close for indefinite periods of times. For those individuals in unhappy and already abusive relationships, the strain caused by these interventions and by having to spend much more time than usual with their live-in partners could create conditions under which more abuse might occur. Both women and men could be victims in this context (Warburton & Raniolo, 2020).

It has been claimed by some researchers in the field that the domestic abuse of men tends not to be as serious as that of women in terms of the injury or harm caused (Mazza et al., 2020). Yet, the actual injury caused, which might be gradable in terms of severity, is not the only relevant measure. Severity is also perceived and this can make the overall harm experienced a matter of subjective judgement on the part of the victim. Data has shown for the United Kingdom that more women (28.4% than men (13.6%) were recorded as having been domestically abused Office for National Statistics, 2019). These figures hide the equally serious factor of the way individual victims experience their abuse. One further finding that sheds more insight on this point was that more women (52%) than men (41%) victims experienced associated emotional and mental problems. Yet, men were more likely to sustain physical injuries from their partners than were women. More men who were victims (4.3%) than women who were victims (0.4%) sustained internal injuries such as broken bones or teeth, from domestic abuse incidents (Office of National Statistics, 2018). Oher kinds of abusive behaviour more often reported for male victims than for female victims included having their spending monitored and controlled, being deprived of food and being deprived of their personal property (Brooks, 2020).

Physically or mentally abusive relationships between intimate partners can take various forms. It can be sexual and non-sexual in nature, but usually involves some form of violence. In most cases, the perpetrators are men and the victims are women, but this can also be reversed. The violence can sometimes spread beyond intimate partners to children in the household. In some cases, the abuse is exclusively between adults and children. Many experts recognised early on in the SARS-COV-2 pandemic that extreme government measures that restricted public behaviour across a wide range of settings could create stressful conditions in households that could in turn ignite abusive relationships. In those households where there was already a catalogue of such incidents, there was an increased probability that they would recur. Reviews of early pandemic evidence on this issue confirmed these collateral risks of societal lockdowns (Mazza et al., 2020).

Children as Victims

The lockdowns during the 2020 coronavirus pandemic resulted in many parents staying home as their workplaces closed and many children being banished to their homes as well as schools closed completely or open only to children or key workers placing both parents and children under strain. For children, the disruption to their school life and education was worrying especially for those studying for critical examinations that would determine their futures. While many continued with their schoolwork at home, some children, especially from poor backgrounds, suffered disproportionately as their homes lacked the space to work in and their families often lacked the technology needed for remote learning. Then, there were variances in the degree to which schools had prepared for this crisis situation. Parents were invited to enjoin with teachers and become home educators for their children. Many parents felt ill-equipped to take on this role. Many also, if they were working from home, lacked the time to play part-time school teacher to their children.

It is therefore understandable that many households felt under considerable psychological pressure and that this could lead to a build-up anxiety, frustration and even anger. Children might experience neglect from their parents and their schools and feel completely at loss as to what to do. Their demands on busy parents could leave tempters frayed. In households where uneasy relationships already existed, these additional pressures created greater risks of aggressive behavioural outbursts (Humphreys et al., 2020; Tronick et al., 2021).

School closures, the disappearance of outdoor pursuits and bans from seeing friends in person together triggered widespread anxiety among children. This, in turn, caused distress in children, disrupted their sleep patterns, made them more irritable than usual such that they became a bigger nuisance to parents already under a lot of pressure of their own from loss of income, trying to help educate their children and coping with keeping the household running under highly constrained circumstances. Households with lone parents could feel under even more strain because a single parent had no other adults with whom to share childcare and home maintenance (Ghosh et al., 2020; Sacco et al., 2020).

Concerns Going Forward

The pandemic created highly unusual living conditions for millions of people that caused much great psychological stress. Anxiety levels across mass publics rose in many parts of the world and created mood states that could also drive potentially harmful behavioural reactions. Sometimes these responses were inward directed and could result in self-harm. On other occasions, they might be outwardly directed and result in harm to others.

One of the biggest impacts of the pandemic was the use by governments of interventions that reduced direct physical and social contact between people. The reason for this was simple. In dealing with a highly infectious and largely airborne disease one of the best ways to control disease transmission was to keep people physically apart as much as possible.

This strategy of disease control through social deprivation created difficult living conditions for many people. Deprived of social contacts on whom they may have depended for psychological support meant that their mental health suffered. Left alone, they lacked coping mechanisms to keep their worries under control. Such effects might be strongly experienced by elderly people many of whom lived alone and were dependent on occasional visits from others. Other elderly lived in care and although not physically alone they may still have looked forward to regular visits from family members. Starved of these contacts, their emotional fragility could lead them to entertain thoughts of self-harm that would be normally kept at bay by their normal social contacts. These reactions were not confined to the elderly. Younger people living on their own could react similarly. Even younger people not living alone might have experienced considerable emotional angst when forced to stay apart from new romantic partners with whom they had not yet lived.

Concerns about increased self-harm behaviour stemmed from observations that the restrictions imposed on most people during the pandemic had created an emotional climate that was known to promote such behaviour among those with relevant predispositions. Evidence had also been obtained from earlier pandemics that showed increased rates of self-harm behaviour, including suicide during those outbreaks. Reassuringly, research across a number of countries indicated no significant changes in suicide rates during the early phases of the pandemic. One study showed that as many as three in ten people said they had entertained suicidal thoughts and around one in ten had attempted suicide, but these figures were not out of line with pre-pandemic comparison data from two earlier periods.

Outwardly directed violence could also be triggered by the stresses caused by pandemic-related restrictions. One area of special concern here was domestic abuse. Heightened pressures caused by the pandemic could also affect people who did not live on their own. These pressures could boil over into interpersonal tensions between people who lived together resulting in violent outbursts. Women and children were the most usual targets or victims of this aggressive behaviour, and men were usually the perpetrators, although this was not invariably the case. Sometimes men could be targets of female aggression.

The relevant psychological pressures could derive from adults and children being kept in close physical proximity for much longer periods than usual. With school and workplace closures, many children and their parents were forced to work from home. This meant spending a lot of time in each other's company during the daytime when they normally would not see each other. Limited workspace at home might be another factor adding to household stress levels. Psychological conditions were therefore created that could cause increased probabilities of violent outbursts. In households in which domestic tensions and abusive behaviour were already established, harmful person-to-person behaviour was especially likely to occur.

The evidence did emerge during the coronavirus pandemic that violence between partners currently living together increased compared with pre-pandemic figures. Violence between former partners not currently living together declined, indicating the impact of stay-at-home rules. This behaviour is often associated with mental health problems among those involved and these problems could be magnified by pandemic-related stress. The restrictions of movement during the pandemic also meant that the normal support services for households experiencing these problems had been suspended. Hence the mitigating forces that might help to calm down volatile domestic settings were missing during the pandemic. Children could also be victims in these settings. Not only might they experience psychological distress from observing violence between their parents or a parent and his/her live-in partner but they might also become direct targets of physical abuse.

One of the most acute concerns was that the pressures that could further catalyse domestic abuse would become more deeply established the longer pandemic-related restrictions were applied. Evidence emerged to indicate that these long-term effects were already being experienced in some countries. Beyond the pandemic, an even greater concern was that these increased occurrences of domestic abuse would not cease immediately after the pandemic, if they had been allowed to persist beyond a critical threshold during it.

References

Appleby, L., Rchards, N., Ibrahim, S., Turnbull, P., Rodway, C., & Kapur, N. (2021). Suicide in England in the COVID-19 pandemic: Early observational data from real time surveillance. *The Lancet*. doi: 10.1016/j.lanepe.2021.100110

Bhavsar, V., Kirkpatrick, K., Calcia, M., & Howard, L. M. (2021). Lockdown, domestic abuse perpetration, and mental health care: gaps in training, research and policy. *The Lancet: Psychiatry*. 8(3): 172–174.

Biswas, T., Scott, J. G., Munir, K., Renzaho, A. M. N., Rawal, L. B., Baxter, J., & Mamun, A. A. (2020). Global variation in the prevalence of suicidal ideation, anxiety and their correlates among adolescents: A population-based study of 82 countries. *EClinicalMedicine*, 24: 100395. doi: 10.1016/j.eclinm.2020.100395

Bradbury-Jones, C., & Isham, L. (2020). The pandemic paradox: the consequences of COVID-19 on domestic violence. *Journal of Clinical Nursing*, 29(13–14): 2047–2049. https://doi.org/10.1111/jocn.15296

Brooks, M. (2020). Male victims of domestic abuse and partner abuse: 50 key facts. Mankind Initiative. Available at: https://www.mankind.org.uk/wp-content/uploads/2020/03/50-Key-Facts-about-Male-Victims-of-Domestic-Abuse-and-Partner-Abuse-March-2020-final.pdf

Brooks, S. K., Webster, R. K., Smith, L. E., et al. (2020). The psychological impact of quarantine and how to reduce it: rapid review of the evidence. *Lancet*, 395(10227): 912–920. doi: 10.1016/S0140-6736(20)30460-8

Bryant, R. A., Gallagher, H. C., Gibbs, L., Pattison, P., MacDougall, C., Harms, L., Block, K., Baker, E., Sinnott, V., Ireton, G., Richardson, J., Forbes, D., & Lusher, D. (2017).Mental health and social networks after disaster. *The American Journal of Psychiatry*, 174(3): 277– 285. doi: 10.1176/appi.ajp.2016.15111403

Calderon-Anyosa, R. J. C., & Kaufman, J. S. (2021). Impact of COVID-19 lockdown policy on homicide, suicide, and motor vehicle deaths in Peru. Preventive Medicine 143: 106331. doi: 10.1016/j.ypmed.2020.106331

Chan, S. M., Chiu, F. K., Lam, C. W., Leung, P. Y., & Conwell, Y. (2006). Elderly suicide and the 2003 SARS epidemic in Hong Kong. *International Journal of Geriatric Psychiatry*, 21(2): 113–118. doi: 10.1002/gps.1432

Coroners Court of Victoria (2020, October 2–5). *Coroners Court Monthly Suicide Data Report*. https://www.coronerscourt.vic.gov.au/sites/default/files/2020-10/Coroners%20Court%20Suicide%20Data%20Report%20-%20Report%202%20-%2005102020.pdf

Courtet, P., Olie, E., Debien, C., & Vaiva, G. (2020). Keep socially (but not physically) connected and carry on: preventing suicide in the age of COVID-19. *Journal of Clinical Psychiatry*, 81(3), 20com13370. doi: 10.4088/JCP.20com13370

Evans, E., Hawton, K., Rodham, K., & Deeks, J. (2005). The prevalence of suicidal phenomena in adolescents: a systematic review of population-based studies. *Suicide & Life-Threatening Behavior*, 35(3): 239–250. doi: 10.1521/suli.2005.35.3.239

Fancourt, D., Bu, F., WanMak, H., & Steptoe, A. (2020). COVID-19 social study. University College London. Retrieved from: https://www.COVIDsocialstudy.org/results

Faust, J. S., Shah, S. B., Du, C., Li, S. X. Lin, Z., & Krumholz, H. M. (2021). Suicide Deaths During the COVID-19 Stay-at-Home Advisory in Massachusetts. March to May 2020. *JAMA network open* 4(1): https://doi.org/10.1001/jamanetworkopen.2020.34273

Gebrewahd, G. T., Gebremeskel, G. G., & Tadess, D. B. (2020). Intimate partner violence against reproductive age women during COVID-19 pandemic in northern Ethiopia 2020: a community-based cross-sectional study. *Reproductive Health*, 17(1): 152. doi: 10.1186/s12978-020-01002-w

Geddes, K., Dziurawiec, S., & Lee, C. W. (2013). Dialectical behaviour therapy for the treatment of emotion dysregulation and trauma symptoms in self-injurious and suicidal adolescent females: a pilot programme within a community-based child and adolescent mental health service. *Psychiatry Journal*, 145219. doi: 10.1155/2013/145219

Ghazinour, M., Mofidi, N., & Richter, J. (2010). Continuity from suicidal ideations to suicide attempts? An investigation in 18–55 years old adult Iranian Kurds. *Social Psychiatry & Psychiatric Epidemiology*, 45(973): 981. doi: 10.1007/s00127-009-0136-z

Ghosh, R., Dubey, M. J., Chatterjee, S., & Dubey, S. (2020). Impact of COVID-19 on children: special focus on the psychosocial aspect. *Minerva Pediatrica*, 72(3): 226–235.

Giussy, B., Facchin, F., Micci, L., Rendiniello, M., Giulini, P., Cattaneo, C., Vercelini, P., & Kuterman, A. (2020). COVID-19, lockdown, and intimate partner violence; Some data from an Italian service and suggestions for future approaches. *Journal of Women's Health*, 29(10): 1239–1242.

Graham-Harrison, E. Giuffrida, A., Smith, H., &c. Ford, E. (2020). Lockdowns Around the World Bring Rise in Domestic Violence. *The Guardian* March 28. Retrieved from: https://www.theguardian.com/society/2020/mar/28/lockdowns-world-rise-domestic-violence

Gunnell, D., Appleby, L., Arensman, E., Hawton, K., John, A., Kapur, N., et al. (2020). Suicide risk and prevention during the COVID-19 pandemic. *Lancet Psychiatry*, 7: 468–471. doi: 10.1016/S2215-0366(20)30171-1

Herrenkohl, T. I., Sousa, C., Tajima, E. A., Herrenkohl, R. C., & Moylan, C. A. (2008). Intersection of child abuse and children's exposure to domestic violence. *Trauma, Violence, Abuse*, 9(2): 84–99. doi: 10.1177/1524838008314797

Hester M., Eisenstadt N., Ortega-Avila A., Morgan K., Walker S., & Bell J. (2019). Centre for Gender and Violence Research, University of Bristol; Bristol: Evaluation of the Drive Project – a three-year pilot to address high-risk, high-harm perpetrators of domestic abuse. Retrieved from: http://driveproject.org.uk/wp-content/uploads/2020/01/Drive-Evaluation-Report-Final.pdf

Holt, N. R., Neumann, J. T., McNeil, J. J., & Cheng, A. C. (2020). Implications of COVID-19 in an ageing population. *Medical Journal of Australia*, 213(8): 342–344.e1. doi: 10.5694/mja2.50785

Humphreys, K. L., Myint, M. T., & Zeanah, C. H. (2020). Increased risk for family violence during the COVID-19 pandemic. *Pediatrics*, 146(1): e20200982. doi: 10.1542/peds.2020-0982

Ivandic, R., & Kirchmaier, T. (2020, 30th June). Home is not a safe place for everyone: domestic abuse between partners increased during lockdown. Retrieved from: https://blogs.lse.ac.uk/covid19/2020/06/30/home-is-not-a-safe-place-for-everyone-domestic-abuse-between-current-partners-increased-during-lockdown/

Ivandic, R., Kirchmaier, T., & Linton, B. (2020). Changing patterns of domestic abuse during COVID-19 lockdown. SSRN. Retrieved from: Ivandic, R., & Kirchmaier, T., & Linton, B. (2020). Changing patterns of domestic abuse during Covid-19 lockdown, CEP Discussion Papers dp1729, Centre for Economic Performance, London School of economics and Political Science, London, UK. Retrieved from: https://ideas.repec.org/p/cep/cepdps/dp1729.html

Joiner, T. (2005). *Why People Die by Suicide*. Harvard University Press.

Klonsky, E. D., May, A. M., & Saffer, B. Y. (2016). Suicide, suicide attempts, and suicidal ideation. *Annual Review of Clinical Psychology*, 12: 307–330. doi: 10.1146/annurev-clinpsy-021815-093204

Lapid, M. I., Koopmans, R., Sampson, E. L., Van den Block, L., & Perisah C. (2020). Providing quality end-of-life care to older people in the era of COVID-19: perspectives from five countries. *International Journal of Psychogeriatrics*, 1–8 [11 May].

Lee, J. (2020). Reflections feature mental health effects of school closures during COVID-19. *Lancet Child and Adolescent Health*, 4: 421. doi: 10.1016/S2352-4642(20)30109-7

Lee, S. J., & Ward, K. P. (2020). Stress and Parenting during the Coronavirus Pandemic. (Research Brief, Parenting in Context Research Lab). Retrieved from: https://www.parentingincontext.org/uploads/8/1/3/1/81318622/research_brief_stress_and_parenting_during_the_coronavirus_pandemic_final.pdf

Lee, S. J., Ward, K. P., Lee, J. Y., & Rodriguez, C. M. (2020). Parental social isolation and child maltreatment risk during the COVID-19 pandemic. *Journal of Family Violence*. Advance publication at: 10.1007/s10896-020-00244-3

Mars, B., Heron, J., Klonsky, E. D., Moran, P., O'Connor, R. C., Tilling, K., Wilkinson, P., & Gunnell, D. (2019). Predictors of future suicide attempt among adolescents with suicidal thoughts or non-suicidal self-harm: a population-based birth cohort study. *The Lancet Psychiatry*, 6(4): 327–337. doi: 10.1016/S2215-0366(19)30030-6

Mazza M., Marano G., Lai C., Janiri L.,& Sani G. (2020). Danger in danger: interpersonal violence during COVID-19 quarantine. *Psychiatry Research*, 289: 113046. doi: 10.1016/j.psychres.2020.113046

Moffitt, P., Aujla, W., Giesbrecht, C. J., Grant, I., & Straatman, A.-L. (2020). Intimate partner violence and COVID-19 in rural, remote, and Northern Canada: Relationship vulnerability and risk. *Journal of Family Violence*, 1–12. doi: 10.1007/s10896-020-00212-x

Neeleman, J., de Graaf, R., & Vollebergh, W. (2004). The suicidal process; prospective comparison between early and later stages. *Journal of Affective Disorders*, 82(1): 43– 52. doi: 10.1016/j.jad.2003.09.005

New Zealand Family Violence Clearinghouse (2020). *Preventing and Responding to family, Whānau and Sexual Violence during COVID-19*. Auckland, NZ: University of Auckland. Retrieved from: https://nzfvc.org.nz/COVID-19/preventing-responding-violence-COVID-19

Nock, M. K., Borges, G., Bromet, E. J., Alonso, J., Angermeyer, M., Beautrais, A., Bruffaerts, R., Chiu, W. T., de Girolamo, G., Gluzman, S., de Graaf, R., Gureje, O., Haro, J. M., Huang, Y., Karam, E., Kessler, R. C., Lepine, J. P., Levinson, D., Medina-Mora, M. E., Ono, Y., ... Williams, D. (2008). Cross-national prevalence and risk factors for suicidal ideation, plans and attempts. *The British Journal of Psychiatry*, 192(2): 98– 105. doi: 10.1192/bjp.bp.107.040113

Norman, A. H. M., Griffiths, M. D., Pervin, S., & Ismail, M. N. (2021). The detrimental effects of the COVID-19 pandemic on domestic violence against women. *Journal of Psychiatric Research*, 134: 111–112.

O'Connor, R. C. (2011). Towards an integrated motivational-volitional model of suicidal behaviour. In R. C. O'Connor, S. Platt, & J. Gordon (Eds.), *International Handbook of Suicide Prevention: Research, Policy and Practice* (pp. 181–198). Wiley Blackwell. doi: 10.1002/9781119998556.ch11

O'Connor, R. C., Wetherall, K., Cleare, S., Eschle, S., Drummond, J., Ferguson, E., O'Connor, D. B., & O'Carroll, R. E. (2018). Suicide attempts and non-suicidal self-harm: National prevalence study of young adults. *British Journal of Psychology Open*, 4(3): 142–148. doi: 10.1192/bjo.2018.14

O'Connor, R., Wetherall, K., Cleare, S., McClelland, H., Melson, A., Niedzwiedz, C., O'Carroll, R. E., O'Connor, D. B., Platt, S., Scowcroft, E., Watson, B., Zortea, T., Ferguson, E., & Robb, K. (2020). Mental health and wellbeing during the COVID-19 pandemic: Longitudinal analyses of adults in the UK COVID-19

Mental Health & Wellbeing study. *The British Journal of Psychiatry*, 1–8. Advance online publication. doi: 10.1192/bjp.2020.212

Office of National Statistics (2018). Appendix tables: Partner abuse in detail – (Tables 9 & 12) *In: Statistics ONS*. Retrieved from: www.ons.gov.uk

Office for National Statistics (2019). Appendix Tables: Domestic Abuse Prevalence and Victim Characteristics (Table 1a) *In: Statistics ONS*. Retrieved from: www.ons.gov.uk

Office of National Statistics (2020). Appendix tables: homicide in England and Wales (Table 10a) *In: Statistics ONS*. Retrieved from: www.ons.gov.uk

Office of National Statistics (2020). Domestic abuse during the coronavirus (COVID-19) pandemic, England and wales, November 2020. Retrieved from: https://www.ons.gov.uk/peoplepopulationandcommunity/crimeandjustice/articles/domesticabuseduringthecoronaviruscovid19pandemicenglandandwales/november2020

Oram S., Trevillion K., Khalifeh H., Feder G., & Howard L. M. (2013a). Systematic review and meta-analysis of psychiatric disorder and the perpetration of partner violence. *Epidemiology and Psychiatric Science*, 23: 361–376.

Oram S., Flynn S. M., Shaw J., Appleby L., & Howard L. M. (2013b). Mental illness and domestic homicide: a population-based descriptive study. *Psychiatric Services*, 64: 1006–1011.

Peterman A., Potts A., O'Donnell M., Thompson K., Shah N., Oertelt-Prigione S., et al. (2020). *Pandemics and Violence Against Women and Children*. Center Global Development Working Paper 528, 2020. Retrieved from: https://www.cgdev.org/publication/pandemics-and-violence-against-women-and-children

Pierce, M., Hope, H., Ford, T., Hatch, S., Hotopf, M., John, A., Kontopantelis, E., Webb, R., Wessely, S., McManus, S., & Abel, K. M. (2020). Mental health before and during the COVID-19 pandemic: a longitudinal probability sample survey of the UK population. *Lancet Psychiatry*, (10): 883–892. doi: 10.1016/S2215-0366(20)30308-4

Pokhrel, S., Sedhai, Y. R., & Atreya, A. (2020). An increase in suicides amidst the coronavirus disease 2019 pandemic in Nepal. *Medicine, Science and the Law*, 61(2): 161–162. doi: 10.1177/0025802420966501

Pokhrel, S., & Chhetri, R. (2021). A Literature Review on Impact of COVID-19 Pandemic on Teaching and Learning. *Higher Education for the Future*, 8(1): 133–141. https://doi.org/10.1177/2347631120983481

Qin, P., & Mehlum, L. (2020). National observation of death by suicide in the first 3 months under COVID-19 pandemic. *Acta Psychiatrica Scandinavica*, 143(1): 92–93. doi: 10.1111/acps.13246

Ribeiro, J. D., Franklin, J. C., Fox, K. R., Bentley, K. H., Kleiman, E. M., Chang, B. P., & Nock, M. K. (2016). Self-injurious thoughts and behaviors as risk factors for future suicide ideation, attempts, and death: a meta-analysis of longitudinal studies. *Psychological Medicine*, 46(2): 225–236. doi: 10.1017/S0033291715001804

Rodriguez, C. M., Lee, S. J., Ward, K. P., & Pu, D. F. (2020). The perfect storm: Hidden risk of child maltreatment during the COVID-19 pandemic. *Child Maltreatment*. doi: 10.1177/ 1077559520982066

Rossi, F. S., Shankar, M., Buckholdt, K., Bailey, Y., Israni, S. T., & Iverson, K. M. (2020). Trying times and trying out solutions: Intimate partner violence screening and support for women veterans during COVID-19. *Journal of General International Medicine*, 35(9): 2728–2731. doi: 10.1007/s11606-020-05990-0

Sacco, M. A., Caputo, F., Ricci, P., Sicilia, F., De Aloe, L., Bonetta, C. F., Cordasco, F., Scalise, C., Cacciatore, G., Zibetti, A., Gratteri, S., & Aquila, I. (2020). The impact of the Covid-19 pandemic on domestic violence: The dark side of home isolation during quarantine. *Medico Legal Journal*, 88(2): 71–73.

Sveticic, J., & De Leo, D. (2012). The hypothesis of a continuum in suicidality: A discussionon its validity and practical implications. *Mental Illness*, 4: e15. doi: 10.4081/mi.2012.e15

Swannell, S. V., Martin, G. E., Page, A., Hasking, P., & St John, N. J. (2014).Prevalence of nonsuicidal self-injury in nonclinical samples: Systematic review, meta-analysis and meta-regression. *Suicide & Life-Threatening Behavior*, 44(3): 273–303. doi: 10.1111/sltb.12070

Tarrier, N., Taylor, K., & Gooding, P. (2008). Cognitive-behavioral interventions to reduce suicide behavior: A systematic review and meta-analysis. Behavior Modification, 32(1), 77–108. https://doi.org/10.1177/0145445507304728

Tochie, J. N., Ofakem, I., Ayissi, G., Endomba, F. T., Fobellah, N. N., Wouatong, C., & Temgoua, M. N. (2020). Intimate partner violence during the confinement period of the COVID-19 pandemic: Exploring the French and Cameroonian public health policies. *Pan-African Medical Journal*, 35(Suppl 2): 54. doi: 10. 11604/pamj.supp.2020.35.2.23398

Tronick, E., Grumi, S., & Provenz, L. (2021). The three-plague nature of COVID-19 pandemic: Implications for women and children and exposure to violence. *Pediatric and Emergency Care*, 37(2): e89–e90.

Tsui V., Cheung M., & Leung P. (2010). Help-seeking among male victims of partner abuse: Men's hard times. *Journal of Community Psychology*, 38(6): 769–780.

Ueda, M., Nordström, R., & Matsubayashi, T. (2020). *Suicide and mental health during the COVID-19 pandemic in Japan. medRxiv 2020* [Preprint.]. doi: 10. 1101/2020.10.06.20207530

Van Gelder N., Peterman A., & Potts A.(2020). COVID-19: reducing the risk of infection might increase the risk of intimate partner violence. *EClinicalMedicine*, 21: 100348. doi: 10.1016/j.eclinm.2020.100348

Van Gelder, N., Peterman, A., Potts, A., O'Donnell, M., Thompson, K., Shah, N., Oertelt-Prigione, S.Gender and COVID-19 Working group (2020). COVID-19: reducing the risk of infection might increase the risk of intimate partner violence. *EClinicalMedicine*, 21: 100348. doi: 10.1016/j.eclinm.2020.100348 Retrieved from: https://www.journals.elsevier.com/eclinicalmedicine

Viero, A., Barbara, G., Montisci, M., Kusterman, K., & Cattaneo, C. (2021). Violence against women in the COVID-19 pandemic: A review of the literature and a call for shared strategies to tackle health and social emergencies. *Forensic Science International*, 319: 110650. doi: 10.1016/j.forsciint.2020.110650

Vu, N. L., Jouriles, E. N., McDonald, R., & Rosenfield, D. (2016). Children's exposure to intimate partner violence: A meta-analysis of longitudinal associations with child adjustment problems. *Clinical Psychology Review*, doi: 10.1016/j.cpr.2016.04.003

Wand, A. P. F., & Perisah, C. (2020). COVID-19 and suicide in older adults: The elephant in the room. *Medical Journal of Australia*, 213(7): 335–335e1. doi: 10. 5694/mja2.50763

Wand, A. P. F., Perisah, C., Draper, B., & Brodaty, H. (2018). Why do the very old self-harm? A qualitative study. *American Journal of Geriatric Psychiatry*, 26: 862–871.

Wand, A. P. F., Zhong, B.-L., Chiu, H. F. K., Draper, B., & De Leo, D. (2020). COVID-19: The implications for suicide in older adults. *International Psychogeriatrics*, 32(10): 1225–1230. doi: 10.1017/S1041610220000770

Warburton, E., & Raniolo, G. (2020). Domestic abuse during COVID-19: What about the boys? *Psychiatry Research*, 291: 113155. doi: 10.1016/j.psychres.2020.113155

WHO (2020). COVID-19 and violence against women what the health sector/system can do? Retrieved from: https://www.who.int/emergencies/diseases/novel-coronavirus-2019/advice-for-public?gclid=EAIaIQobChMI-Nz4_crs6QIVwQ0rCh1P_glUEAAYASACEgIe4PD_BwE

Wildeman, C., Emanuel, N., Leventhal, J. M., Putnam-Hornstein, E., Waldfogel, J., & Lee H. (2014). The prevalence of confirmed maltreatment among US children, 2004 to 2011. *JAMA Pediatrics*, 168(8): 706–713. doi: 10.1001/jamapediatrics.2014.410

Windsor, T. D., Curtis, R. G., & Luszcz, M. A. (2015). Sense of purpose as a psychological resource for aging well. *Developmental Psychology*, 51(7): 975–986. doi: 10.1037/dev0000023

Yu, R., Nevado-Holgado, A. J., & Molero, Y. (2020). Mental disorders and intimate partner violence perpetrated by men towards women: A Swedish population-based longitudinal study. *PLoS Medicine*, 16(12): e1002995. doi: 10.1371/journal.pmed.1002995

Zapor, H., Wolford-Clevenger, C., & Johnson, D. M. (2015). The association between social support and stages of change in survivors of intimate partner violence. *Journal of Interpersonal Violence*, 33(7): 1051–1070.

Chapter 9

Lockdown and Alcohol Consumption

Among the biggest public health challenges faced by many societies are the health consequences of excessive consumption of alcoholic drinks. If alcohol misuse develops into a chronic behaviour over time, it can increase the risk of heart disease and cancer and disrupt family relationships and performance at work (Keyes et al., 2011) As the pandemic progressed, data emerged of increased alcohol sales (Colbert et al., 2022; Rehm et al., 2020). Drinking excessive alcohol during a national health crisis caused by a highly infectious disease is unwise because it weakens the immune system and might therefore render someone more susceptible to serious illness if they became infected (Clay & Parker, 2020; Koob et al. 2021; Rehm et al., 2020).

One further unhelpful side effect would be individuals with serious alcohol-related problems presenting themselves at hospitals when hospital resources were already stretched dealing with COVID-19 cases (Balhara et al., 2020; Narasimha et al., 2020; Smalley & Cisarik, 2020). Alcohol-related mental health problems could also catalyse pandemic-related anxieties leading to extreme responses including suicide attempts (Dsouza et al., 2020). Evidence emerged also that elevated alcohol levels were found in nearly three in ten people hospitalised for COVID-19 in England (Hamer et al. 2020).

Past experience had shown that alcohol consumption levels do appear to be sensitive to times of great crisis. Studies of public reactions following episodes of extreme terrorism, natural catastrophes and pandemics have confirmed this observation (DiMaggio et al., 2009; Goncalves et al., 2020). Such events can create widespread public distress which, in turn, gives rise to mental health impacts. With more prevalent anxiety and expression, the scene is set for some people to turn to alcohol (Ramalho, 2020).

Pandemics and Alcohol Consumption

It is worth pausing to review key findings that related to pre-COVID crises because they provide an important interpretive context for analysing behaviour changes and intervention impacts during the 2020 pandemic.

DOI: 10.4324/9781003274377-9

Greater exposure to the terrorist attacks on the US incidents of 9/11 were found to have impacted some groups of people hard. Among the outcomes were higher rates of binge drinking were detected among them, and especially among young male adults with higher levels of education and with posttraumatic stress disorders (Murphy et al., 2007; Welch et al., 2014, 2017; Yu et al., 2016). There were also higher levels of hospitalisation for alcohol-related or drug-related problems over many years afterwards (Hirst et al., 2018).

Economic crises, such as those experienced in 2008, could also increase levels of stress and anxiety across populations and especially in those directly affected by these events. The latter included people working in the finance sector and those whose businesses suffered or who lost their homes. Some people turned to alcohol as a coping mechanism. Drinking to excess however simply piles on another stressor which undermines mental and physical health and well-being (Karanikolos et al., 2013; Ásgeirsdóttir et al., 2014; de Goeij et al., 2015).

Research in the United States found a decline in overall population consumption of alcohol after the 2008 financial crisis but also increased binge drinking in specific population sub-groups. Most especially, white, less well-educated, unemployed, young adult males were most likely to display heavy drinking bouts (Bor et al., 2013; de Goeij et al., 2015; Kaplan et al., 2016; Yang et al., 2018; Kalousova & Burgard, 2014; Brown et al., 2019). Thus, in general, economic stressors have been linked to excessive drinking. The pandemic, of course, was a massive economic stressor.

The Potential for Increased Alcohol Consumption

The COVID-19 pandemic gave rise to economic, physical and mental health concerns. There were more focused worries also about specific behavioural changes that flowed from these broader issues, including changes in people's alcohol consumption (Callinan et al., 2021; Callinan et al., 2021; Pollard et al., 2020). The research into alcohol consumption, however, is characterised by wide variations in methodologies and quality and the findings therefore have not been always consistent.

Some studies from Europe and North America revealed that both general alcohol consumption and heavy drinking increased during the pandemic compared with pre-pandemic. There were studies conducted in Australia, Belgium, France and the United States that showed increased drinking during the pandemic (Pollard et al., 2020; Roland et al., 2020; Vanderbruggen et al., 2020; Callinan et al., 2021). Other evidence emerged from Latin America and the Caribbean that alcohol consumption dropped during the pandemic (Pan-American Health Organization, 2020).

The findings could have been affected by a failure to differentiate between buying for future home consumption and buying on licensed premises for immediate consumption (Rolland et al., 2020; Vanderbruggen et al., 2020; Callinan et al., 2021). The latter, of course, was largely banned for large swathes of time during the pandemic because bars, clubs and restaurants were all closed. For some people therefore, more drinking at home could have been compensation for not being allowed to drink in licensed premises. Open-ended and in-depth interviews with further revealed that some people were drinking more at home during the pandemic than they did before it started (Nicholls & Conroy, 2021; Vandenberg et al., 2021).

Various indicators of alcohol consumption were used to measure consumption volume during the pandemic. These included measures of sales volumes, amount of duty collected and self-reports from people questioned in surveys about their drinking habits. Data on volume sales of alcohol products in the United Kingdom that compared pre-pandemic with pandemic levels showed a 25% increase in sales levels (Public Health England, 2021). Similar findings emerged for the United States where retail sales of alcohol products increased by around one-fifth from 2019 to 2020 (Castaldelli-Maia et al., 2021).

Consumer purchases of alcohol outside of licensed premises increased across the pandemic, rising by over 24% from 2019–2020 to 2020–2021. When asking people directly to estimate whether their volume of alcohol consumption had changed during the pandemic, most felt it had not changed and among the remainder, similar proportions said it had increased or decreased. Many polls that asked people to estimate their personal consumption levels were poor in quality and so many have provided imprecise measures of what was going on. Evidence did emerge that while average levels of drinking may not have changed that much, problematic alcohol consumption did increase (by +59%) from March 2020 to March 2021 in the United Kingdom. Further reinforcing this finding, it was also noted that alcohol-related hospitalisations increased in 2020 compared with 2019 (+3%) (Public Health England, 2021).

The 2020 Pandemic and Alcohol Consumption

During the pandemic, a circular relationship could evolve in which the restrictions on public behaviour encouraged some people to drink more and this response then put them at greater risk of ill-health both from excessive alcohol intake and also by weakening their immune system and rendering them more susceptible to serious illness from COVID-19 infection. Turning to alcohol to cope with the stress caused by the pandemic might have alleviated the pressure on people in the short term, but more generally, it could also have put them at greater health risk over time (Calina et al., 2021).

Survey evidence from the United States indicated that alcohol consumption levels rose during 2020, compared with 2019, among people aged

30–80 years. Americans in general were estimated to have drunk around 14% more alcohol over this time, and women exhibited a 17% increase in consumption. On examining the propensity of women to consume for drinks or more in a single session, this behaviour increased by a substantial 41% in 2020 compared with 2019 (Pollard et al., 2020)

A study in Poland followed through respondents' drinking habits from pre-pandemic to during the pandemic and found that while most people said they did not change their drinking habits during the pandemic, three in ten (30%) did change. The latter were approximately evenly split between those saying they had drunk more (14%) and those saying they had drunk less (16%). Those who said they had drunk more during the pandemic tended to be younger than those who said they had reduced their drinking. Those who increased their drinking were also those who displayed psychological characteristics and mental symptoms that would have predicted this behaviour (Chodkiewicz et al., 2020).

A small United Kingdom survey found that 17% of respondents said they had drunk more alcohol than they usually did during the lockdown. Those with poorer mental health tended to show the greatest increases in drinking behaviour (Jacob et al., 2020). Another United Kingdom survey found that 15% of respondents said they had been drinking more in reach sessions during lockdown (The Lancet Gastroenterology, 2020).

A large Belgian survey revealed increased alcohol consumption during the pandemic. Being younger, less well-educated and out of work were associated with this behaviour and it also appeared to be motivated by boredom, social isolation, loss of a daily routine and loneliness (Vanderbruggen et al., 2020).

In contrast, a further Belgian investigation found that two-thirds of the students questioned in that country (68%) reported reduced alcohol consumption during lockdown compared with before it. Under one in five (17%) said they had been drinking more during the lockdown. Some students were already heavy drinkers before lockdown and they had identified motives such as social confidence building and stress coping as reasons for their drinking behaviour. Those heavy drinkers driven by social motives before lockdown reported reduced drinking during it (Bollen et al., 2021). Where drinking represented a crutch to help individuals cope with everyday stresses, it could increase among those who felt even more stressed during the pandemic (Evans et al., 2021).

Further evidence of increased alcohol consumption emerged from other parts of Europe, Australia and China (Panagiotidis et al., 2020; Sidor & Rzymski, (2020).

In the United Kingdom, an investigation of alcohol consumption patterns through sales figures rather than self-reports indicated that alcohol purchases did not increase substantially during the January to July period which overlapped with the first pandemic lockdown compared to the same period each year from 2015 to 2018 (Anderson et al., 2020). In Australia, another approach to measuring alcohol use was to measure the level of alcohol in wastewater during quarantine periods. The data showed a reduction in levels of alcohol indicating less consumption. One reason for this was probably the removal of opportunities to drink in bars, clubs and restaurants and far fewer household social events (Bade et al., 2020). There was also a drop in alcohol consumption by college students once university campuses had closed and many students returned home to their parents (Bade et al., 2020; White et al., 2020).

Further evidence emerged that the pandemic triggered more drinking especially when people found themselves spending more time at home. Causes included boredom, disruption of normal routines and stress (Nanos Research, 2020), many people drank because they were sad and feeling down (Fiocruz, 2020). This elevated alcohol drinking was particularly likely to occur when individuals were quarantined and totally confined to their homes, not being allowed to go out at all (Sidor & Rzymski, 2020).

Being made unemployed and then stuck at home with the children (whose schools had closed) were connected to increased alcohol consumption. The loss of regular daily routines and structures, with the end unknown, meant that some people struggled to find a purpose in life. With the loss also of their social contacts, people were limited in the social network support they could call upon and this only served to put them under greater stress (Vanderbruggen et al., 2020).

In some countries, such as Australia, evidence emerged of reported alcohol consumption reaching dangerous levels among over half of people surveyed during the early phases of the pandemic (Newby et al., 2020; Stanton et al., 2020). This pattern was most pronounced among young people aged 18–25 among whom alcohol consumption became progressively more problematic, the more stressed they felt (Callinan et al., 2020).

In China, as well, research coming out of Hubei, where the pandemic is widely believed to have started, revealed signs of harmful alcohol use that exceeded that observed in other Chinese provinces (Ahmed et al., 2020). In Wuhan, the city at the epicentre of the initial outbreak, there were widespread reports from people of feeling stressed. Women drinkers as well as men drinkers displayed the highest stress levels, which were considerably higher than those reported among teetotallers (Zhang et al., 2020). Other findings indicated an increased prevalence of negative coping strategies, which included excess alcohol consumption, among people experiencing general psychological malaise (Lee, 2020; Liang et al., 2020).

Population Subgroups and Variances in Alcohol Consumption during the Pandemic

In examining changes in alcohol-related behaviour during the pandemic, it is relevant to ask whether some people were more susceptible to these effects than others. Once again, the empirical evidence was not always consistent. In general, though, it would seem that all kinds of people were affected by the pandemic in ways that triggered more drinking. There were no consistent patterns to this behaviour change, at least in respect of demographic-level differences. Both men and women, the young and the old, and individuals from different occupations and socio-economic strata could be susceptible. It was clear that specific life experiences during the pandemic such as being required to work from home with limited space to do so, reduce income or job loss, could aggravate a person's mental state in ways that might encourage them to turn to alcohol as a coping mechanism.

Mental health status was known to be linked to drinking problems anyway and plenty of evidence emerged during the pandemic that enhanced population-wide worries about the crisis and its impact on people's own lives created the social and psychological conditions that could promote alcohol abuse (Callinan et al., 2021; Evans et al., 2021; Goncalves et al., 2020; Lechner et al., 2020).

Gender-Related Differences

Women and men have been found to show different orientations towards alcohol. While much attention has been directed towards alcohol abuse among men, it is also prevalent among women. One consistent finding has been that women are more likely than men to turn to drink when under severe emotional distress (Kuntsche et al., 2014; Guinle & Sinha, 2020). During the pandemic, the emotional stresses that were known to be caused by public behaviour restrictions were hypothesised to have a bigger impact on women than on men (Popay & Williams, 1996; Liu et al., 2015). Hence, potentially, women could have been seen as being at greater risk of collateral damage from pandemic-related restrictions as expressed via the misuse of alcohol (Biddle et al., 2020; Meagher et al., 2020).

Women around the world reported more health-related worries than did men during the pandemic. Women displayed higher rates of clinical anxiety than did men during this period especially if they had dependent children living with them (Palsson et al., 2020). Evidence from the United States showed an increase in drinking days (+14%) during the pandemic compared with a year earlier. The increase was somewhat bigger than this for women (+17%) and greater still for adults aged 30–59 years (+19%) (Pollard et al., 2020).

In Australia, among 14% of people that claimed to have increased their consumption during the pandemic compared with just before it, this claim was more prevalent among women (18%) than men (11%). Further survey evidence from the same country indicated that a bigger percentage of women (32%) than of men (23%) claimed to have increased their drinking. Pre-pandemic data had shown that women were only about half as likely as men to drink risky amounts of alcohol. During the pandemic, however, their alcohol consumption reports suggested that they had reacted worse than men and this might have been because they were harder hit than were men, on average, by the mental strain of coping during this crisis (Sanderson et al., 2020).

Modest rates of increased alcohol consumption were detected in one Canadian study, with just 12% of those surveyed saying they had increased their drinking. Emotional distress triggered by the pandemic was associated with increased consumption, but no differences were found between women and men in their relative propensities to drink more, even though women generally reported more emotional stress responses to the pandemic (Thompson et al., 2021).

A pan-European survey that covered 21 countries and 31,000+ respondents who were surveyed from April to July 2020 indicated a general decrease in alcohol consumption during the initial phases of the pandemic, largely explained by a reduction in heavy drinking episodes and no differences between men and women in terms of amounts of alcohol consumption (Kilian et al., 2021).

Survey evidence that is reliant on self-reports of behaviour, expressed in simplified formats and often only on one occasion, may not reflect the nature of people's orientation towards alcohol. Across the pandemic, psychological reactions did not remain unchanging. Initial responses in terms of alcohol consumption could quite easily change as the pandemic and its associated restrictions on public behaviour wore on. Qualitative research evidence produced by a study with Australian women revealed that their initial reactions to the pandemic did not immediately modify their orientations towards alcohol but that over time these changed for some of the women who turned to alcohol to help them get through the pandemic. Although the women in this study recognised the health risks of alcohol consumption when interviewed before the pandemic, during it, as their lifestyles changed so too did their risk assessments. For women that had previously been cautious about drinking, the stresses of the pandemic and associated social distancing led some to temporarily suspend their concerns as they used alcohol as a coping mechanism for the more immediate crisis of the pandemic (Lunnay et al., 2021).

Age-Related Differences

Research conducted with young adults, the age group most likely to go out drinking socially, found mixed results in terms of whether the pandemic triggered changes in normal drinking amounts. While the locations of drinking were forced to change when governments closed licensed premises such as bars, clubs and restaurants, whether or not people then went out and drank more at home was not a foregone conclusion. Under the most extreme lockdown conditions, people from different households were not allowed to meet up. Internationally, research emerged to show both increased and decreased amounts of consumption based on self-reports (Bollen et al., 2021; Charles et al., 2021; Evans et al., 2021; Lechner et al., 2020; Ryerson et al., 2021; Villaneuva et al., 2021).

One Spanish study with young adults recorded no changes in overall reported amounts of alcohol consumption from before the onset of the pandemic and a year after its onset, but there was evidence that those respondents who displayed signs of greater depression were less likely than others to reduce their drinking rates (del Valle Vera et al., 2021).

While mixed evidence emerged during the pandemic that young adults changed their drinking habits, British research indicated an upswing in high-risk drinking among middle-aged people with fewer than one in five (19%) having reported problematic alcohol consumption levels in 2016–2018 and one in four (25%) doing so during the early stages of the pandemic in May 2020. The average reported frequency of four or more drinking episodes per week doubled from 13% to 26% (Daly & Robinson, 2021).

Much of the evidence concerning young people's alcohol drinking habits during the pandemic derived from studies of university students. They were put under considerable pressure by the closure of campuses and most face-to-face classes. Remote tuition was offered instead, but some universities were better prepared than others for this switch to a different learning platform. Some evidence emerged that changed living circumstances caused by pandemic-related restrictions, especially among students living away from their parents for the first time, triggered more alcohol consumption (Ryerson et al., 2021).

As seen from the evidence reviewed, some studies found conflicted results for different sections of the populations they sampled. Others found that drinking appeared to increase on one measure of consumption and decrease on another. One study of American college students, for example, found that they reported a decrease in the number of drinks consumed per week, but also more frequent drinking episodes (White et al., 2020). Other studies showed that young people were actually more likely than older age groups to decrease how much alcohol they drank during the pandemic (Callinan et al., 2021; Chodkiewicz et al., 2020). There could be a conformity effect at play here with most students indicating that neither they nor their friends had felt it necessary to drink more during these exceptional circumstances (Graupensperger et al., 2021).

Further evidence emerged from a relatively small-scale sample of students ($n = 312$) that they reported drinking less after their university campus had been closed and that this was reflected in the number of drinks that they consumer per week and the maximum amount they consumed in any given day. There was some evidence of a marginal increase in the number of days on which they drank in the average week. Further analysis revealed, however, two distinct groups. Those students that returned home to live with their parents after campus closure drank far less than usual, while those that remained on campus with their peers during this period actually reported more frequent drinking (White et al., 2020).

Reasons for Increased Alcohol Consumption

The economic impact of the pandemic caused considerable stress for many people whose jobs and businesses were threatened. On top of this, the social isolation and general lack of structured activities, with most services and public spaces being closed, triggered extreme boredom in many. When this happens, people look around for things to do and under pandemic lockdown conditions, the options were limited. Drinking therefore provided a convenient form of escapism (Struk et al., 2020). The desperation to alleviate boredom might also encourage people to seek out less constructive solutions to their psychological concerns. This means that if they find an answer in alcohol, it is less likely to be a measured reaction under these extreme life conditions (Struk et al., 2020). There can then be a circularity in the harm that emerges from this non-constructive behaviour. Social distancing might encourage more drinking and more drinking might in turn trigger more social distancing breaches as drinkers seek to meet up and ignore the rules (Suffoletto et al., 2020).

Whether individuals increased or decreased their consumption of alcohol during the pandemic might also have depended on how they had responded psychologically to the crisis more generally. Those people who experienced increased stress during the pandemic, perhaps because of the threat it posed to their employment or simply because of the loss of normal daily structure to their lives were more likely to report greater use of alcohol (Grossman et al., 2020; Neill et al., 2020; Schmits & Glowacz, 2021). For others, loss of income and the financial stress it caused led to them buying and therefore consuming less alcohol (Vanderbruggen et al., 2020). Further evidence is examined below concerning psychological substrates to changes in alcohol consumption behaviour.

While the closure of universities caused many students a lot of distress around the world, there was some reassuring evidence that despite being worried about temporary suspension of normal learning activities, when universities did return to some semblance of normality, many students anxiety responses returned to pre-pandemic levels (Charles et al., 2021)

The pandemic was found to cultivate maladaptive behaviours among young people. Research from Canada indicated that there was less binge drinking among adolescents but signs that drinking had nonetheless become more frequent. Customarily, adolescents preferred to drink socially with their friends. During the pandemic, this socialising was banned and more lone drinking was found to occur. There was further evidence of increased drinking at home with their parents (Dumas et al., 2020).

Adolescents also used their ingenuity to find alternative solutions to prohibitions on normal socialising. They used communication technologies to maintain links with their friends. Face-to-face drinking in the same physical space may have been banned for a time, but face-to-face drinking over a video link was permitted. Many teens turned to this substitute for purely solitary drinking (Dumas et al., 2020).

Mental Health as a Precursor to Greater Alcohol Consumption

Pre-pandemic research had already established that the abuse of alcohol was often linked to mental health problems. Although this was not always true, it was known that individuals experiencing chronic anxiety states or depression would sometimes turn to alcohol as a coping mechanism. Given the potentially stressful circumstances of the pandemic, it might have been expected that the prevalence of mental health problems would increase (Clay & Parker, 2020). As earlier reviewed evidence in this book showed, there were plenty of signs that this did happen. One pattern that did emerge was that if alcohol consumption had increased among individuals, it formed part of a wider syndrome that might also include losing your job, having your education interrupted, experiencing more pressure at home with more people being around than usual, eating more than usual, experiencing disturbed sleep and feeling generally anxious (Son et al., 2020; Tran et al., 2020).

Evidence emerged that the effects of pandemic-associated anxiety could trigger other behaviour changes in the consumption of alcohol quite quickly. One American study found that college students showed signs of increased drinking within the first few weeks of campus closure. Furthermore, those that reported experiencing anxiety or depression symptoms also reported the biggest increase in alcohol intake (Lechner et al., 2020).

Another US study reported that increased alcohol consumption (which included drinking more, drinking excessively with greater frequency and drinking alone) were associated with reports of being depressed. Such effects were found among some samples to kick-in within weeks of pandemic-related behavioural restrictions being imposed (McPhee et al., 2020).

In a US survey of people aged 26–49 years (84% female), six in ten (60%) reported increased pandemic drinking and 13% said they had drunk less than usual during the pandemic. One-third (34%) reported engaging in binge drinking during the pandemic period. Taking into account gender, ethnicity, age and household income, heavier and more frequent drinking were predicted by more reported COVID-related stress, greater availability of alcohol and boredom (Grossman et al., 2020).

A survey of over 13,000 people conducted in 33 countries across the Caribbean and Latin America examined changes in alcohol consumption behaviours during the pandemic compared with pre-pandemic. The researchers used multivariate statistical analyses to identify key predictors of increased alcohol intake. Two-thirds of respondents (65%) identified as alcohol consumers in 2019 said they had engaged in heavy drinking episodes during the COVID-19 pandemic. However, more drinkers said they drank heavily less often during the pandemic (33%) than aid they drank heavily more often (14%). Drinkers drank more heavily more often during the pandemic if they were male and had a higher income and lived in countries that deployed a higher level of quarantine practices.

Other factors that represented *decreased* risks of increased heavy drinking episodes were being unemployed, being a student and living in a household with children. More anxious people also tended to report increased drinking episodes. This research therefore found that specific indigenous characteristics and living circumstances represented pre-existing indicators or drivers of alcohol consumption (Valente et al., 2021).

In an international study, covering 83 countries, increases in alcohol consumption were frequently found among people who had been quarantined. This behaviour shift was especially likely to occur among older people, those who were essential workers, those with children, and those who had a close personal relationship with someone who was seriously ill with COVID-19. Greater personal anxiety and depression and greater impulsivity were also associated with increased pandemic drinking (Sallie et al., 2020).

Lessons Learned

During times of national crisis when the public is confronted with great uncertainty, people understandably become anxious about current threats and concerned about what the future might hold once the crisis is over. Such reactions had been observed with disasters, emergencies and threatening incidents in recent history. They were seen again during the COVID-19 pandemic. Under these psychological conditions, many people will seek coping strategies. Simply suffering unpleasant circumstances is intolerable and unacceptable for many. When this type of situation is experienced therefore people either seek to find solutions to their uncertainty or distractions that take their minds off it. The first approach would generally be regarded as the more constructive way forward. The second might also be constructive but could so easily not be.

Considering what we might expect in terms of pandemic-related effects on alcohol consumption, there can be reasons for people to increase or decrease how much they drink. Pandemic-related stress might drive some people towards greater amounts of drinking as a coping mechanism, especially if they are regular or heavy drinkers already. Then, the reduction in income and loss of jobs through the impact of the pandemic might mean that some people would be unable to afford to drink as much as they might normally drink (Pollard et al., 2020; Rehm et al., 2020).

There was evidence from some research that heavy drinkers prior to the pandemic may have been more likely than more moderate drinkers to increase their intake during the pandemic. Then other evidence emerged to contradict this finding. United Kingdom government analysis investigated where there were differences in changes to alcohol-related behaviour related to habitual pre-pandemic levels of drinking. A sample of alcohol consumers was divided into quintiles based on the volume of alcohol they bought during the two years prior to the first United Kingdom national lockdown. The heaviest pre-pandemic consumers of alcohol exhibited the biggest pandemic increases in alcohol purchases. Those in the heaviest alcohol purchasing quintile accounted for a disproportionate amount of the total increase (42%). Overall, though, most people showed no significant change in how much alcohol they purchased during the pandemic and among those that did, they were more or less equally split between those reportedly drinking more and those reportedly drinking less (Gov.UK. 2021).

Despite concerns that greater stress during the pandemic might encourage heavier drinking, further research among people in the United Kingdom showed that the proportion of people engaging in at-risk levels of drinking fell from pre-pandemic (36%) to during the pandemic (32%). Those turning to drink to cope were people that experienced higher than average levels of anxiety and depression during the pandemic and who had low coping resilience. Loss of job or income did not appear to drive greater reliance on alcohol when soundings were taken in March and July 2020 (McBride et al., 2021).

A study of Portuguese students monitored the behaviour of identified binge drinkers and non-binge drinkers before the pandemic, during it and afterwards. Interestingly, binge drinkers decreased how much they drank during the lockdown and afterwards. Regular binge drinkers exhibited drinking patterns more aligned with infrequent binge drinkers. No evidence emerged that the propensity to engage in binge drinking was related to anxiety or stress levels (Vasconcelos et al., 2021).

Elsewhere, data from Africa, Asia, Europe, North and South America revealed decreases in binge drinking in different time periods in 2020 compared with equivalent time periods in 2019 (Ammar et al., 2020).

Canadian research found several risk factors associated with increased alcohol consumption during the pandemic. These factors included living with children aged under-18, less social connectedness, loss of income and also being depressed. Living alone was also a predictor of increased lone drinking (Wardell et al., 2020). The researchers called for a greater understanding of the way alcohol drinking was used as a coping mechanism during the pandemic in order to devise alternatives that were less threatening to health. There was some evidence that people that already have problems with alcohol or drink habitually were the ones most likely to turn to it as a coping mechanism during the pandemic. Often, excessive consumption of alcohol has been linked back to other mental health problems (Cooper, 1994, Cooper et al., 1995). If drinking as a coping mechanism has become an established behaviour (Merrill et al., 2014; Stevenson et al., 2019), it was likely to surface again during the COVID-19 pandemic.

Pre-established drinking habits could pre-determine how people used alcohol during the pandemic. Hence, pre-COVID binge drinkers were more likely to binge during the pandemic than were pre-COVID moderate drinkers. Further, the more established binge drinkers also suffered from other mental health problems such as depression, the worse their pandemic drinking behaviour was likely to become (Weerakoon et al., 2020).

This chapter has considered public coping choices in relation to COVID-19 and the behavioural restrictions implemented by their governments in response to it specially in relation to their use of alcohol. Moderate drinkers who maintained their habits might have recovered some solace from the pleasure of imbibing. People who turned to drink more seriously during the pandemic could be causing self-harm. Research conducted during the pandemic showed that while there was evidence that some people reported increased alcohol consumption, many others reduced their consumption. Although reducers may not have given up completely, many did report overindulging less often or maintaining only a moderate among of drinking.

References

Ahmed M. Z., Ahmed O., Aibao Z., Hanbin S., Siyu L., & Ahmad A. (2020). Epidemic of COVID-19 in China and associated Psychological Problems. *Asian Psychiatric Journal*, 51: 102092. doi: 10.1016/j.ajp.2020.102092

Ammar A., Brach M., Trabelsi K., Chtourou H., Boukhris O., Masmoudi L., Bouaziz B., Bentlage E., How D., Ahmed M., Müller P., Müller N., Aloui A., Hammouda O., Paineiras-Domingos L. L., Braakman-Jansen A., Wrede C., Bastoni S., Pernambuco C. S., Mataruna L., Taheri M., Irandoust K., Khacharem A., Bragazzi N. L., Chamari K., Glenn J. M., Bott N. T., Gargouri F., Chaari L., Batatia H., Ali G. M., Abdelkarim O., Jarraya M., Abed K. E., Souissi N., Van Gemert-Pijnen L., Riemann B. L., Riemann L., Moalla W., Gómez-Raja J., Epstein M., Sanderman R., Schulz S. V., Jerg A., Al-Horani R., Mansi T., Jmail M., Barbosa F., Ferreira-Santos F., Šimunič B., Pišot R., Gaggioli A., Bailey S. J., Steinacker J. M., Driss T., & Hoekelmann A. (2020). Effects of COVID-19 home confinement on eating behaviour and physical activity: Results of the ECLB-COVID19 international online survey. *Nutrients*, 12: 1583.

Andersen, L. H., Fallesen, P., & Bruckner, T. A. (2021). Risk of stress/depression and functional impairment in Denmark immediately following a COVID-19 shutdown. *BMC Public Health*, 21: 984.

Anderson P., Llopis E. J., O'Donnell A., & Kaner E. (2020). Impact of COVID-19 confinement on alcohol purchases in Great Britain: Controlled interrupted time-series analysis during the first half of 2020 compared with 2015-2018. *Alcohol Alcohol*, 56(3): 307–316. doi: 10.1093/alcalc/agaa128

Ásgeirsdóttir T. L., Corman H., Noonan K., Ólafsdóttir P., & Reichman N. E. (2014). Was the economic crisis of 2008 good for Icelanders? Impact on health behaviors. *Economics and Human Biology*, 13: 1–19. doi: 10.1016/j.ehb.2013.03.005

Avery, A. R., Tsang, S., Seto, E. Y., & Duncan, G. E. (2020). Stress, anxiety, and change in alcohol use during the COVID-19 pandemic: Findings among adult twin pairs. *Frontiers in Psychiatry*, 11: 571084. doi: 10.3389/fpsyt.2020.571084

Bade, R., Simpson, B. S., Ghetia, M., Nguyen, L., White, J. M., & Gerber, C. (2020). Changes in alcohol consumption associated with social distancing and self-isolation policies triggered by COVID-19 in South Australia: a wastewater analysis study. *Addiction*, 116(6): 1600–1605. doi: 10.1111/add.15256

Balhara, Y. P. S., Kattula, D., Singh, S., Chukkali, S., & Bhargava, R. (2020). Impact of lockdown following COVID-19 on the gaming behavior of college students. *Indian Journal of Public Health*, 64(Supplement): S172–S176. doi: 10.4103/ijph.IJPH_465_20

Biddle, N., Edwards, B., Gray, M., & Sollis, K. (2020). *Alcohol Consumption During the COVID-19 Period: May 2020*. Canberra, ACT: ANU Centre for Social Research and Methods; Australian National University.

Bollen, Z., Pabst, A., Creupelandt, C., Fontesse, S., Lannoy, S., Pinon, N., & Maurage, P. (2021). Prior drinking motives predict alcohol consumption during the COVID-19 lockdown: A cross-sectional online survey among Belgian college students. *Addictive Behavior*, 115: 106772.

Bor J., Basu S., Coutts A., Mckee M., & Stuckler D. (2013). Alcohol use during the great recession of 2008–2009. *Alcohol Alcohol*, 48: 343–348. doi: 10.1093/alcalc/agt002

Brown R. L., Richman J. A., Moody M. D., & Rospenda K. M. (2019). Alcohol-related effects of POST-9/11 discrimination in the context of the great recession: Race/ethnic variation. *Addictive Behaviour*, 93: 154–157. doi: 10.1016/j.addbeh.2019.01.019

Calina, D., Hartung, T., Mardare, I., Mitroi, M., Poulas, K., Tsatsakis, A., Rogoveanu, I., & Docea, A. O. (2021). COVID-19 pandemic and alcohol consumption: Impacts and interconnections. *Toxicology Reports*, 8: 529–535.

Callinan, S., & MacLean, S. (2020). COVID-19 makes a stronger research focus on home drinking more important than ever. *Drug and Alcohol Review*, 39(6): 613–615. doi: 10.1111/dar.13125

Callinan, S., Mojica-Perez, Y., Wright, C. J. C., Livingston, M., Kuntsche, S., Laslett, A. M., Room, R., & Kuntsche, E. (2021). Purchasing, consumption, demographic and socioeconomic variables associated with shifts in alcohol consumption during the COVID-19 pandemic. *Drug and Alcohol Review*, 40(2): 183–191. doi: 10.1111/dar.13200

Callinan S., Smit K., Mojica-Perez Y., D'Aquino S., Moore D., & Kuntsche E. (2020). Shifts in alcohol consumption during the COVID-19 pandemic: early indications from Australia. *Addiction*, 116(6): 1381–1399. doi: 10.1111/add.15275 [Epub ahead of print].

Callinan, S., Smit, K., Mojica-Perez, Y., D'Aquino, S., Moore, D., & Kuntsche, E., (2021). Shifts in alcohol consumption during the COVID-19 pandemic: Early indications from Australia. *Addiction*, 116(6): 1381–1388. doi: 10.1111/add.15275

Castaldelli-Maia, J. M., Segura, L. E., & Martins, S. S. (2021). The concerning increasing trend of alcohol beverage sales in the U.S. during the COVID-19 pandemic [published online ahead of print, 2021 Jul 8]. *Alcohol*, 96: 37–42. doi: 10.1016/j.alcohol.2021.06.004

Charles, N. E., Strong, S. J., Burns, L. C., Bullerjahn, M. R., & Serafine, K. M. (2021). Increased mood disorder symptoms, perceived stress, and alcohol use among college students during the COVID-19 pandemic. *Psychiatry Research*, 296: 113706. doi: 10.1016/j.psychres.2021.113706

Chodkiewicz, J., Talarowska, M., Miniszewska, J., Nawrocka, N., & Bilinski, P. (2020). Alcohol consumption reported during the COVID-19 pandemic: The initial stage. *International Journal of Environmental Research and Public Health*, 17: 4677. doi: 10.3390/ijerph17134677

Clay, J. M. & Parker, M. O. (2020). Alcohol use and misuse during the COVID-19 pandemic: A potential public health crisis? *Lancet Public Health*, 5: e259. doi: 10.1016/S2468-2667(20)30088-8

Colbert, G. B., Venegas-Vera, A. V., & Lerma, E. V. (2022). Utility of telemedicine in the COVID-19 era. Reviews of Cardiovascular Medicine, 21(4): 583–587. doi: 10.31083/j.rcm.2020.04.188.

Cooper, M. L. (1994). Motivations for alcohol use among adolescents: Development and validation of a four-factor model. *Psychological Assessment*, 6(2): 117–128. doi: 10.1037/1040-3590.6.2.117

Cooper, M. L., Frone, M. R., Russell, M., & Mudar, P. (1995). Drinking to regulate positive and negative emotions: a motivati onal model ofalcohol use. *Journal of Personality and Social Psychology*, 69(5): 990–1005. doi: 10.1037//0022-3514. 69.5.990

de Goeij, M. C. M., Suhrcke, M., Toffolutti, V., van de Mheen, D., Schoenmakers, T. M., & Kunst, A. E. (2015). How economic crises affect alcohol consumption and alcohol-related health problems: A realist systematic review. *Social Science and Medicine*, 131: 131–146. doi: 10.1016/j.socscimed.2015.02.025

Daly, M., & Robinson, E. (2021). Psychological distress and adaptation to the COVID-19 crisis in the United States. *Journal of Psychiatric Research*, 136, 603–609. https://doi.org/10.1016/j.jpsychires.2020.10.035

del Valle Vera, B., Carmona-Marquez, J., Lozano-Rojas, O. M., Parrado-Gonzalez, A., Vidal-Gine, C., Pautassi, R. M., & Fernandez-Calderon, F. (2021). Changes in alcohol use during the COVID-19 pandemic among young adults: The prospective effect of anxiety and depression. *Journal of Clinical Medicine*, 10(19): 4468. doi: 10.3390/jcm10194468

DiMaggio, C., Galea, S., & Li, G. (2009). Substance use and misuse in the aftermath of terrorism. A Bayesian meta-analysis. *Addiction*, 2009(104): 894–904. doi: 10.1111/j.1360-0443.2009.02526.x

Dsouza, D. D., Quadros, S., Hyderabadwala, Z. J., & Mamun, M. A. (2020). Aggregated COVID-19 suicide incidences in India: Fear of COVID-19 infection is the prominent causative factor. *Psychiatry Research*, 290: 113145. doi: 10.1016/ j.psychres.2020.113145.

Dumas, T. M., Ellis, W., & Litt, D. M. (2020). What does adolescent substance use look like during the COVID-19 pandemic? Examining changes in frequency, social contexts, pandemic-related predictors. *Journal of Adolescent Health*, 67: 354–361. doi: 10.1016/j.jadohealth.2020.06.018

Evans, S., Alkan, E., Bhangoo, J. K., Tenenbaum, H., & Ng-Knight, T. (2021). Effects of the COVID-19 lockdown on mental health, wellbeing, sleep, and alcohol use in a UK student sample. *Psychiatry Research*, 298: 113819.

Fiocruz. (2020). Available online at: https://convid.fiocruz.br/index.php?pag= bebiba_alcoolica (accessed 16 June 2020).

Goncalves, P. D., Moura, H. F., Abrantes do Amaral, R., Castaldelli-Maia, J. M., & Malbergier, A. (2020). Alcohol use and COVID-19: Can we predict the impact of the pandemic on alcohol use based on the previous crisis in the 21st century? A brief review. *Frontiers in Psychiatry*, 11: 581113. doi: 10.3389/fpsyt.2020. 581113

Gov.U. K. (2021, 15th July) Monitoring alcohol consumption and harm during the COVID-19 pandemic: summary. Retrieved from: https://www.gov.uk/government/ publications/alcohol-consumption-and-harm-during-the-covid-19-pandemic/ monitoring-alcohol-consumption-and-harm-during-the-covid-19-pandemic-summary

Graupensperger, S., Jaffe, A. E., Fleming, C. N., Kilmer, J. R., Lee, C. M., & Larimer, M. E. (2021). Changes in college student alcohol use during the COVID-19 pandemic: Are perceived drinking norms still relevant? *Emerging Adulthood*. doi: 10.1177/2167696820986742

Grossman, E. R., Benjamin-Neelon, S. E., & Sonneenschein, S. (2020). Alcohol consumption during the COVID-19 pandemic: A cross-sectional survey of US adults. *International Journal of Environmental Research and Public Health*, 17(24): 9189. doi: 10.3390/ijerph17249189

Guinle, M. I. & Sinha, R. (2020). The role of stress, trauma and negative affect in alcohol misuse and alcohol use disorder in women. *Alcohol Research*, 40(2): 05. doi: 10.35946/arcr.v40.2.05

Hamer, M., Kivimäki, M., Gale, C. R., & Batty, G. D. (2020). Lifestyle risk factors, inflammatory mechanisms, and COVID-19 hospitalization: A community-based cohort study of 387,109 adults in UK. *Brain, Behavior, and Immunity*, 87: 184–187. https://doi.org/10.1016/j.bbi.2020.05.059

Henderson, E. (2021, 19th August) Study shows an increase in home drinking during COVID-19 pandemic. Medical Life Sciences news. Retrieved from: https:// www.news-medical.net/news/20210819/Study-shows-an-increase-in-home-drinking-during-COVID-19-pandemic.aspx

Hirst A., Miller-Archie S. A., Welch A. E., Li J., & Brackbill R. M. (2018). Post-9/11 drug- and alcohol-related hospitalizations among world trade center health registry enrollees, 2003-2010. *Drug and Alcohol Dependency*, 187: 55–60. doi: 10.1016/j.drugalcdep.2018.01.028

Jacob L., Smith L., Armstrong N. C., Yakkundi A., Barnett Y., Butler L., Mcdermott D. T., Koyanagi A., Shin J. I., Meyer J., Firth J., Remes O., López Sánchez G. F., & Tully M. A. (2020). Alcohol use and mental health during COVID-19 lockdown: A cross-sectional study in a sample of UK adults. *Drug and Alcohol Dependency*, 219: 108488. doi: 10.1016/j.drugalcdep.2020. 108488

Kalousova L. & Burgard S. A. (2014). Unemployment, measured and perceived decline of economic resources: contrasting three measures of recessionary hardships and their implications for adopting negative health behaviors. *Social Science Medicine*, 106: 28–34. doi: 10.1016/j.socscimed. 2014.01.007

Kaplan, M. S., Huguet, N., Caetano, R., Giesbrecht, N., Kerr, W. C., & McFarland, B. H. (2016). Heavy Alcohol Use Among Suicide Decedents Relative to a Nonsuicide Comparison Group: Gender-Specific Effects of Economic Contraction. *Alcoholism: Clinical and Experimental Research*, 40(7): 1501–1506. https://doi.org/10.1111/acer.13100

Karanikolos M., Mladovsky P., Cylus J., Thomson S., Basu S., Stuckler D., et al. (2013). Financial crisis, austerity, and health in Europe. *Lancet*, 381: 1323–1331. doi: 10.1016/S0140-6736(13)60102-6

Keyes, K. M., Hatzenbuehler, M. L., & Hasin, D. S. (2011). Stressful life experiences, alcohol consumption, and alcohol use disorders: the epidemiologic evidence for four main types of stressors. *Psychopharmacology*, 218(1): 1–17. https://doi.org/10.1007/s00213-011-2236-1

Kilian, C., Rehm, J., Allebeck, P., Braddick, F., Gual, A., Bartak, M., Bloomfield, K. Gil, A., Neufeld, M., O'Donnell, A., et al., (2021). Alcohol consumption during the COVID-19 pandemic in Europe: a large-scale cross-sectional study in 21 countries. *Addiction*. Retrieved from: 10.1111/add.15530

Koob, C., Schröpfer, K., Coenen, M., Kus, S., & Schmidt, N. (2021). Factors influencing study engagement during the COVID-19 pandemic: A cross-sectional study among health and social professions students. *PLOS ONE*, 16(7): e0255191. https://doi.org/10.1371/journal.pone.0255191

Kuntsche, E., Gabhainn, S. N., Roberts, C., Windlin, B., Vieno, A., Bendtsen, P., Hublet, A., Tynjälä, J., Välimaa, R., Dankulincová, Z., Aasvee, K., Demetrovics, Z., Farkas, J., van der Sluijs, W., de Matos, M. G., Mazur, J., & Wicki M. (2014). Drinking motives and links to alcohol use in 13 European countries. *Journal in Studies of Alcohol and Drugs*, 75(3): 428–437.

Lechner, W. V., Laurene, K. R., Patel, S., Anderson, M., Grega, C., & Kenne, D. R. (2020). Changes in alcohol use as a function of psychological distress and social support following COVID-19 related University closings. *Addictive Behavior*, 110: 106527.

Lee, S. A. (2020). How much "Thinking" about COVID-19 is clinically dysfunctional? *Brain, Behaviour and Immunity*, 87: 97–98. doi: 10.1016/j.bbi.2020.04.067

Liang, L., Ren, H., Cao, R., Hu, Y., Qin, Z., Li C., et al. (2020). The effect of COVID-19 on youth mental health. *Psychiatry Quarterly*, 91: 841–852. doi: 10. 1007/s11126-020-09744-3

Liu, Y., Nguyen, N., & Colditz, G. A. (2015). Links between alcohol consumption and breast cancer: A look at the evidence. *Women's Health*. (2015) 11: 65–77. doi: 10.2217/WHE.14.62

Lunnay, B., Foley, K., Meyer, S. B., Warin, M., Wilson, C., Olver, I., Miller, E. R., Thomas, J., & Ward, P. R. (2021). Alcohol consumption and perceptions of health risks during COVID-19: A qualitative study of middle-aged women in South Australia. *Frontiers in Public Health*, 9: 616870. doi: 10.3389/fpubh.2021. 616870

Meagher, N., Carpenter, L., Marinkovic Chavez, K., Vasileva, M., MacDougall, C., Gibbs, L., et al. (2020). *Distancing Measures in the Face of COVID-19 in Australia: Summary of National Survey Findings.* Melbourne, VIC: Melbourne School of Population and Global Health, University of Melbourne. Retrieved from: https://mspgh.unimelb.edu.au/__data/assets/pdf_file/0010/3641770/2020-Annual-Report_spread.pdf

Merrill, J. E., Wardell, J. D., & Read, J. P. (2014). Drinking Motives in the Prospective Prediction of Unique Alcohol-Related Consequences in College Students. *Journal of Studies on Alcohol and Drugs,* 75(1): 93–102. https://doi.org/10.15288/jsad.2014.75.93

McBride, O., Bunting, E., Harkin, O., Butter, S., Shevlin, M., Murphy, J., Mason, L., Hartman, T. K., McKay, R., Hyland, P., Levita, L., Gibson-Miller, J., Bennett, K. M., Stocks, T. V. A., Martinez, A., Vallières, F., & Bentall, R. P. (2021). Testing both affordability-availability and psychological-coping mechanisms underlying changes in alcohol use during the COVID-19 pandemic. *PLoS ONE,* 17(3): e0265145. ISSN 1932-6203

McPhee, M. D., Keough, M. T., Rundle, S., Heath, L. M., Wardell, J. D., & Hendershot C. S. (2020). Depression, environmental reward, coping motives and alcohol consumption during the COVID-19 Pandemic. *Frontiers in Psychiatry,* 11: 574676. Published 2020 Oct 30. doi: 10.3389/fpsyt.2020.574676

Murphy J., Brackbill R. M., Thalji L., Dolan M., Pulliam P., & Walker D. J. (2007). Measuring and maximizing coverage in the world trade centre health registry. *Statistics in Medicine,* (2007) 26: 1688–1701. doi: 10.1002/sim.2806

Nanos Research (2020). *Canadian Centre on Substance and Addiction* (2020). Available online at: https://www.ccsa.ca/sites/default/files/2020-06/CCSA-NANOS-Increased-Alcohol-Consumption-During-COVID-19-Report-2020-en_0.pdf (accessed 14 June, 2020).

Narasimha, V. L., Shukla, L., Mukherjee, D., Menon, J., Huddar, S., Panda, U. K., Mahadevan, J., Kandasamy, A., Chand, P. K., Benegal, V., & Murthy, P. (2020). Complicated Alcohol Withdrawal—An Unintended Consequence of COVID-19 Lockdown. *Alcohol and Alcoholism,* 55(4): 350–353. doi: 10.1093/alcalc/agaa042

Neill, E., Meyer, D., Toh, W. L., van Rheenen, T. E., Phillipou, A., Tan, E. J., & Rossell, S. L. (2020). Alcohol use in Australia during the early days of the COVID-19 pandemic: Initial results from the COLLATE project. *Psychiatry and Clinical Neuroscience,* 74: 542–549.

Newby J., O'Moore K., Tang S., Christensen H., & Faasse K. (2020). Acute mental health responses during the COVID-19 pandemic in Australia. *PloS one,* 15(7): e0236562. https://doi.org/10.1371/journal.pone.0236562

Nicholls, E. & Conroy, D. (2021). Possibilities and pitfalls? Moderate drinking and alcohol abstinence at home since the COVID-19 lockdown. *International Journal of Drug Policy,* 88: 103025. doi: 10.1016/j.drugpo.2020.103025

Palsson, O., Ballou, S., & Gray, S. (2020). *The U.S. National Pandemic Emotional Impact Report.* Durham, NC: UNC Medical School and Cambridge MA: Harvard Medical School. Retrieved from: https://www.pandemicimpactreport.com/report/PalssonBallouGray_2020_PandemicImpactReport.pdf

Panagiotidis P., Rantis K., Holeva V., Parlapani E., and Diakogiannis I. (2020). Changes in alcohol use habits in the general population, during the COVID-19 lockdown in Greece. *Alcohol and Alcohol*, 55: 702–704.

Pan-American Health Organization (2020). Alcohol use during the COVID-19 pandemic in Latin America and the Caribbean. Retrieved from: https://www.paho.org/en/node/73607

Pollard M. S., Tucker J. S., & Green H. D., Jr (2020). Changes in adult alcohol use and consequences during the COVID-19 pandemic in the US. *JAMA Network Open*, 3: e2022942–e2022942.

Popay, J. & Williams, G. (1996). Public health research and lay knowledge. *Social Science and Medicine*, 42: 759–768. doi: 10.1016/0277-9536(95)00341-X

Public Health England (2021, 15th July). Monitoring alcohol consumption and harm during the COVID-19 pandemic: summary. Retrieved from: https://www.gov.uk/government/publications/alcohol-consumption-and-harm-during-the-covid-19-pandemic/monitoring-alcohol-consumption-and-harm-during-the-covid-19-pandemic-summary

Ramalho, R. (2020). Alcohol consumption and alcohol-related problems during the COVID-19 pandemic: A narrative review. *Australas. Psychiatry*, 28: 524–526.

Rehm, J., Kilian, C., Ferreira-Borges, C., Jernigan, D., Monteiro, M., Parry, C. D., Sanchez, Z. M., & Manthey, J. (2020). Alcohol use in times of the COVID 19: Implications for monitoring and policy. *Drug and Alcohol Review*, 39: 301–304.

Rolland, B., Haesebaert, F., Zante, E., Benyamina, A., Haesebaert, J., & Franck, N. (2020). Global changes and factors of increase in caloric/salty food intake, screen use, and substance use during the early COVID-19 Containment Phase in the General Population in France: Survey study. *JMIR Public Health Surveillance*, 6(3): e19630. doi: 10.2196/19630 Erratum in: JMIR Public Health Surveillance, 2021 Jul 20; 7(7): e31906.

Ryerson, N. C., Wilson, O. W., Pena, A., Duffy, M., & Bopp, M. (2021). What happens when the party moves home? The effect of the COVID-19 pandemic on US college student alcohol consumption as a function of legal drinking status using longitudinal data. *Translational Behavioral Medicine*, 11: 772–774.

Sallie, S. N., Ritou, V., Bowden-Jones, H. & Voon, V. (2020). Assessing international alcohol consumption patterns during isolation from COVID-19 pandemic using an online survey: Highlighting negative emotionality mechanisms. Multicenter Study, *BMJ Open*, 10(11): e44276. doi: 10.1136/bmjopen-2020-044276

Sanderson, W. C., Arunagiri, V., Funk, A. P., Ginsburg, K. L., Krychiw, J. K., Limowski, A. R., Olesnycky, O. S., & Stout, Z. (2020). The Nature and Treatment of Pandemic-Related Psychological Distress. *Journal of Contemporary Psychotherapy*, 50(4), 251–263. https://doi.org/10.1007/s10879-020-09463-7

Schmits, E., & Glowacz, F. (2021). Changes in alcohol use during the COVID-19 pandemic: Impact of the lockdown conditions and mental health factors. *International Journal of Mental Health and Addiction*, 4th January, 1–12. doi: 10.1007/s11469-020-00432-8

Sepulveda-Loyola, W., Rodriguez-Sanchez, I., Perez-Rodriguez, P., Ganz, F., Torralba, R., Oliveira, D. V., & Rodriguez-Manas, L. (2020). Impact of social isolation due to COVID-19 on health in older people: Mental and physical effects and recommendations. *Journal of Nutrition, Health and Aging*, 24(9): 938–947. doi: 10.1007/s126-3-020-1469-2

Sidor A. & Rzymski P. (2020). Dietary choices and habits during COVID-19 lockdown: Experience from Poland. *Nutrients*, 12: 1657.

Smalley, D. & Cisarik, P. M. (2020). COVID-19 experience 2020: Changes in the Laboratory Environment. *Medical Research Archives*, 8(10). https:journals.kei.org/index.php/mra

Son, C., Hegde, S., Smith, A., Wang, X., & Sasangohar, F. (2020). Effects of COVID-19 on college students' mental health in the United States: Interview survey study. *Journal of Medical Internet Research*, 22: e21279

Stanton R., To Q. G., Khalesi S., Williams S. L., Alley S. J., Thwaite T. L., et al. (2020). Depression, anxiety and stress during COVID-19: Associations with changes in physical activity, sleep, tobacco and alcohol use in Australian adults. *International Journal of Environmental Research and Public Health*, 17: 4065. doi: 10.3390/ijerph17114065

Stevenson, J. C., Millings, A., & Emerson, L. M. (2019). Psychological well-being and coping: the predictive value of adult attachment, dispositional mindfulness, and emotion regulation. *Mindfulness*, 10, 256–271. https://doi.org/10.1007/s12 671-018-0970-8.

Struk A. A., Scholer A. A., Danckert J., & Seli P. (2020). Rich environments, dull experiences: how environment can exacerbate the effect of constraint on the experience of boredom. *Cognition and Emotion*, 34: 1517–1523. doi: 10.1080/ 02699931.2020.1763919

Suffoletto B., Ram N., & Chung T. (2020). In-person contacts and their relationship with alcohol consumption among young adults with hazardous drinking during a pandemic. *Journal of Adolescent Health*, 67: 671–676. doi: 10.1016/j.jadohealth. 2020.08.007

The Lancet Gastroenterology (2020). H Drinking alone: COVID-19, lockdown, and alcohol-related harm. *Lancet Gastroenterology and Hepatology*, 5: 625–625.

Thompson, K., Dutton, D. J., MacNabb, K., Liu, T., Blades, S., & Asbridge M. (2021). Changes in alcohol consumption during the COVID-19 pandemic: Exploring gender differences and the role of emotional distress. *Health Promotion and Chronic Disease Prevention in Canada*, 41(9): 254–263. English, French. doi: 10.24095/hpcdp.41.9.02

Tran, T. D., Hammarberg, K., Kirkman, M. Nguyen, H. T. M., & Fisher, J. (2020). Alcohol use and mental health status during the first months of COVID-19 pandemic in Australia. *Journal of Affective Disorders*, 277: 810–813.

Valente, J. Y., Sohi, I., Garcia-Cerde, R., Monteiro, M. G., & Sanchez, Z. M. (2021). What is associated with the increased frequency of heavy episodic drinking during the COVID-19 pandemic? Data from the PAHO regional web-based survey. *Drug and Alcohol Dependence*, 221: 108621. doi: 10.1016/ j.drugalcdep. 2021.108621

Vandenberg, B., Livingston, M., & O'Brien, K. (2021). When the pubs closed: Beer consumption before and after the first and second waves of COVID-19 in Australia. *Addiction*, 116(7): 1709–1715. doi: 10.1111/add.15352

Vanderbruggen, N., Matthys, F., Van Laere, S., Zeeuws, D., Santermans, L., Van den Ameele, S., & Crunelle, C. L. (2020). Self-reported alcohol, tobacco, and Cannabis use during COVID-19 lockdown measures: Results from a web-based survey. *European Journal of Addiction Research*, 26(6): 309–315. doi: 10.1159/ 000510822

Vasconcelos, M., Crego, A., Rodrigues, R., Almeida-Antunes, N., & López-Caneda E. (2021). Effects of the COVID-19 mitigation measures on alcohol consumption and binge drinking in college students: A longitudinal survey. *International Journal of Environmental Research and Public Health*, 18(18): 9822. doi: 10.3390/ijerph181 89822

Villanueva, V. J., Motos, P., Isorna, M., Villanueva, V., Blay, P., & Vázquez-Martínez, A. (2021). Impacto de las medidas de confinamiento durante la pandemia de Covid-19 en el consumo de riesgo de alcohol. *Revista Espanola de Salud Pública*, 95: e1–e13

Wardell, J. D., Kempe, T., Rapinda, K. K., Single, A., Bilevicius, E. M. Frohlich, J. R., Hendershot, C. S., & Keough, M. T. (2020). Drinking to cope during COVID-19 pandemic: The role of external and internal factors in coping motive pathways to alcohol use, solitary drinking and alcohol problems. *Alcoholism: Clinical and Experimental Research*, 44(10): 2073–2083.

Weerakoon, S. M., Jetelina, K. K., & Knell, G. (2020). Longer time spent at home during COVID-19 pandemic is associated with binge drinking among US adults. *American Journal of Drug and Alcohol Abuse*, 1–9. doi: 10.1080/00952990.2020. 1832508

Welch, A. E., Caramanica, K., Maslow, C. B., Cone, J. E., Farfel, M. R., Keyes, K. M., et al. (2014). Frequent binge drinking five to six years after exposure to 9/11: Findings from the World Trade Center health registry. *Drug and Alcohol Dependency*, 140: 1–7. doi: 10.1016/j.drugalcdep.2014.04.013

Welch, A. E., Caramanica Zweig, K., McAteer, J. M., & Brackbill, R. M. (2017). Intensity of binge drinking a decade after the September 11th terror attacks among exposed individuals. *American Journal of Preventive Medicine*, 52: 192–198. doi: 10.1016/j.amepre.2016.10.034

White, H. R., Stevens, A. K., Hayes, K., & Jackson, K. M. (2020). Changes in alcohol consumption among college students due to COVID-19: Effects of campus closure and residential change. *Journal of Studies in Alcohol and Drugs*, 81: 725–730

Yang, C., Potts, R., & Shanks, D. R. (2018). Enhancing learning and retrieval of new information: a review of the forward testing effect. *npj Science of Learning*, 3, 8. https://doi.org/10.1038/s41539-018-0024-y

Yu, S., Considine, K., Saleska, E., Walker, D., Richards, A., Nguyen, M., et al. (2016). New York City department of health and mental hygiene, RTI international. In: *World Trade Center Health Registry Wave 4 Survey: Data File User's Manual*. New York, NY: World Trade Center Health Registry.

Zhang, Y., Wang, J., Zhao, J., Tanimoto, T., Ozaki, A., Crump, A., et al. (2020). Association between quarantined living circumstances and perceived stress in Wuhan City during the COVID-19 outbreak: A rapid, exploratory cross-sectional study. *SSRN [preprint]*. doi: 10.2139/ssrn.3556642

Chapter 10

Lockdown and Gambling Behaviour

Among the potentially damaging side-effects of the 2020 SARS-CoV-2 pandemic were reports that problem gambling rates were increasing. The MP for Swansea East, Carolyn Harris, claimed that social distancing restrictions and the closure of all leisure and entertainment amenities meant that many people had become bored and had also been saving money because there was less to spend it on and so had taken to gambling, which could be done online from home to fill time and amuse themselves (Wells, 2020). With most people's lives being put on hold online entertainment had become a bigger business. Public mental health had suffered and, in their desperation, many people were searching for some respite from the anxiety caused by the pandemic and the stimulus deprivation caused by the government's interventions (Holmes et al., 2020; Torales et al., 2020). Online gambling was available on tap 24/7 and there were concerns that established gamblers might bet more often and non-gamblers might try it out and get hooked.

With the closure of sports events and gambling outlets such as betting shops and casinos, many customary gambling opportunities were suspended for an indefinite period. In response, the gambling industry expanded their online operations. The market had already been moving in that direction and had established a wide range of types of gambling on websites that included lotteries and all kinds of casino games. In the online world, many of the companies behind these games were based outside the countries whose gamblers they served. This meant that they operated under different jurisdictions and this could result in games being played in ways that local regulations would normally have outlawed (SBC News, 2020). Some jurisdictions had become so anxious about the possible negative effects of online gambling – given its constant availability and the ease with which money could be staked – that they imposed limits on stakes to protect players (*The Guardian*, 2020).

Online Gaming and COVID-19 – Initial Concerns

The "stay-at-home" instructions issued to their populations by many governments as the 2020 pandemic infiltrated their borders and spread

DOI: 10.4324/9781003274377-10

dramatically across the population isolated people on a mass scale. Some people coped with these restrictions better than others. They created the psychological conditions that triggered anxiety and depression in some and also promoted problem behaviour among those predisposed to show it. This included gambling behaviour. Most people who gamble occasionally do not have a problem. Even during the pandemic, they may have turned to gambling a little more often than usual as a time-filler and distraction. For individuals who on the evidence of their past behaviour could be classed as being at least moderately at risk or high risk from gambling because they could allow it to control them rather than the other way around, the isolation caused by the pandemic presented a potentially greater problem. Extended periods of being stuck at home and unable to go out and meet family and friends not only meant they had more spare time on their hands, but they were also bored. Gambling for such people might be an obvious coping mechanism (King & Delfabbro, 2020).

Evidence emerged during the pandemic, from quite early on, that many people increased their consumption of digital entertainment. For many, this may have comprised increased use of film and TV streaming services, but for some also it took the form of online gaming and online gambling (Perez, 2020). One major communications business in the United States reported a substantial (75%) increase in online gaming activity following the introduction of stay-at-home directives from public health authorities (Pantling, 2020). A major increase in internet traffic was reported in Italy which was hit hard by the pandemic and whose government deployed very severe lockdown restrictions (Lepido & Rolander, 2020). Indeed, the online gaming industry initially worked with health authorities, including the World Health Organization (WHO), in encouraging people to play online games as a respite from the boredom of extreme lockdowns (Abel & McQueen, 2020). The WHO even launched a social media campaign called "Play Apart Together" that encouraged people to comply with social isolation advice but to find remote activities for personal amusement (Ghebreyesus, 2020; Maden, 2020).

Further evidence had emerged that online gambling could result in more gamblers getting into debt than offline gambling. With offline gambling, players often had to go out of their way to leave home and go to specific venues where gambling took place – such as betting shops, casinos and sports venues. Many of these outlets were not open all the time. This was not true of online gambling which provided 24/7 availability and gamblers did not even have to leave home (Wood & Williams, 2011; Gainsbury, 2015). Gambling via mobile phone interfaces also meant that gamblers could place bets from any location at any time.

Under these extreme circumstances, online gaming was regarded as playing a socially positive role in continuing to keep people occupied and connected to others and safely. Earlier campaigns involving online gaming had been found to produce positive results (Granic et al., 2014) and does not have to be problematic (Király et al., 2017). This type of remote activity was found to be useful as an antidote to loneliness (Carras et al., 2017) which had become a major issue for many people during the pandemic. It was certainly better for people than other less healthy, but not uncommon coping behaviours such as consuming more alcohol, increased rug use or over-eating (Corbin et al., 2013; Razzoli et al., 2017).

Despite these gaming initiatives during the pandemic, there is also a body of research showing that increased amounts of game playing beyond an optimal threshold can be a risk factor for various psychological side-effects. Playing these games excessively can pose risk to physical and mental health (Saunders et al., 2017; King et al., 2019). Over-reliance on gaming can disrupt other aspects of life, including normal social interaction and for children and adolescents, it might also disrupt schoolwork. The social distancing restrictions deployed during the 2020 pandemic opened up opportunities for gaming behaviour as a time filler. Extended periods of lockdown in which most people seldom left their homes could have driven some people towards reliance on this particular online activity especially where it was readily available throughout the day.

One longer-term worry was that if youngsters became dependent upon online gaming for long enough during the pandemic, this behaviour could be strongly conditioned to the point where it would persist even after lockdown restrictions were lifted. To counter this possibility, it is important that players diversify their diet of online gaming and from time to time engage with games that focus on social connections that might even be carried over into the physical world (Addiction Policy Forum, 2020).

Some initial evidence showed modest changes only in gambling behaviours in Europe in 2020 (Håkansson et al., 2020). As the pandemic progressed, evidence emerged that some switching between types of gambling did occur. Gamblers who gambled in casinos, for example, switched to online casino gambling but tended to engage in less intense gambling in that context. One study of Swiss casino users found a little over half (55%) said they had played online casino games during lockdown (Lischer et al., 2021). This shift to online gambling both for regular offline gamblers and others new to gambling raised concerns about wider possible harms emanating from gambling (Håkansson et al., 2020; Horner, 2020).

Gambling Volumes based on Industry Data

Much of the research that investigated the gambling-related side-effects of the pandemic relied upon self-reports from people questioned in surveys. Industry data that measure player traffic in both offline and online gambling environments and the revenues generated from this activity represent other measures of gambling behaviour that are not reliant on inconsistent and subjective memories of people about their own gambling behaviour.

The closure of all major sports events that triggered much gambling immediately stripped away from a significant proportion of gambling opportunities that were highly popular with gamblers (Håkansson et al., 2020). Some countries took action to control the potential migration of gamblers from offline to online betting and game playing amidst fears that online gambling could be more problematic because of the ease with which it could be played from home (*The Guardian*, 2020). Self-report evidence had indicated early on that sports-related gambling must have been affected by the impact of pandemic-related restrictions as reports of doing it collapsed while reports of engaging with online gambling games displayed a distinct upswing (Håkansson, 2020a, 2020b).

Swedish evidence based on taxation revenues showed an initial decrease in the amount of online gambling activity, including online casino betting, but this shift stabilised after a few months. Similarly, horse betting increased at first but then returned with months to pre-pandemic levels. The initial evidence for the first months of the pandemic in Sweden indicated that the big gambling brands saw an upturn in business but the smaller ones experienced a downturn in revenues. Overall, then, some offline sports betting activities disappeared and the businesses built upon them experienced loss of revenues. Over time, however, it was less clear whether overall amounts of gambling had actually changed much as a result of the pandemic (Håkansson, 2020c).

Consumer data for Great Britain from March to November 2020 indicated no sustained changes in overall gambling activity but there were some shifts in specific types of betting. There was evidence that there had been progressively increased interest in online gambling but that this did not mean that all gamblers were gambling more than normal. There was a small increase (3%) in active online accounts and also in the volume of bets (4%). Overall, gross gambling yield increased by 13 per cent. There was an increase in online slot-machine gambling in terms of numbers of bets placed and amount of betting income these yielded. Numbers of gambling sessions did not increase, but average length of the gambling session did (from 1 minute to 22 minutes). This reinforces the observation that people were looking for ways of entertaining themselves and many people had more time on their hands because of the impact of lockdown. Such evidence did raise concerns that this behaviour needed to be monitored (The Gambling Commission, 2021).

Brown and Hickman (2020) examined gambling trends in Australia during March and April 2020 and found that the prevalence of online gambling declined across these two months as did the proportions of those who engaged in online betting and reported any online gambling from March (60%) to April (46%). While opportunities to gamble decreased by a small margin across these two months, more respondents said they had gambled more money in April (33%) than in March (20%). Those most likely to report increased spending on gambling in April (but not in March) were male, aged under-40 and lived as a couple with children.

A national population survey in Sweden (9% of whom were problem gamblers) found that a small proportion (4%) reported increased pandemic gambling. Indeed, increases in online gambling were noted most for online casino games, online horse betting and online lotteries. Overall betting was down for sports events more generally. Increased gambling was also more likely to occur among people with a history of problem gambling and among those who drank more alcohol (Håkansson, 2020c). If gambling did take a significant upturn in numbers betting and average stake sizes this opens up further risks of increased rates of problem gambling with all the known mental health side-effects this can bring (Håkansson et al., 2020).

Behavioural scientists have come to regard gambling as potentially "addictive" (Potenza et al., 2019). Problem gambling is no small issue with one estimate calculating that it affected between one and five per cent of the world's population (SBC News. (2020). The pandemic presented an unprecedented state of affairs for governments, public health services and people around the world. Prior evidence had provided indications however that major national crises could trigger increased interest in gambling. One example of this occurred after the 2008 financial crisis and another occurred specifically in Greece after its own economic problems with the European Union (*The Guardian*, 2020). Financial hardship can drive increased playing of lotteries, for example (Håkansson, 2020a; Reuters, 2020). While casino gambling might drop away when times are hard, buying lottery tickets does not (Håkansson, 2020b).

While financial hardship might motivate some people to take up gambling in the belief that a stroke of good luck will solve their problems, another factor at play during a pandemic is boredom. When confronted with a highly infectious new disease for which no medical treatments or immunisation is available, governments have conventionally resorted to other measures and these often entail restrictions on public behaviour. In 2020, most countries locked down significant parts of their economies and in doing so also restricted the amount of social interaction between people. Many people were confined to their homes and had no opportunities to socialise with others or find entertainment outside the home. This created ideal conditions for those so inclined to indulge in gambling (King et al., 2020).

There was some evidence also that some types of online gambling increased as those who would normally have placed bets on sports events could not do this because these events had been suspended. Yet, sports betting did not stop completely. Fresh opportunities for this type of gambling were provided by betting companies by inviting gamblers to place bets on teams playing in leagues that would not normally be covered by the media – either from overseas or from minor domestic leagues (Brown & Hickman, 2020). There were stories of gamblers creating their own betting scenarios (*Financial Times*, 2020), but mostly they transferred their interest from one conventional betting scenario to another. Overall, however, only a minority of sports bettors made this type of activity switch, but among them, the great majority was classified as moderate to high-risk problem gamblers.

Sports betting virtually disappeared at the outset of the pandemic because most sporting events stopped. There were fairly modest amounts of shifting to online casino betting as a substitute (Auer et al., 2020; Lindner et al., 2020). While offline and live sports betting experienced a slump as pandemic-related restrictions started to bite and the events with which this betting was associated was suspended, online betting volumes remained buoyant. The latter behaviour was maintained by the popularity of non-sports online gambling games that were not reliant on live sports events. Other early pandemic findings indicated that most of the observed increased amounts of gambling once COVID-19 had become established occurred among problem gamblers (Håkansson, 2020b).

Self-Reported Changes in Gambling Behaviour

Even before the pandemic, research has emerged to show that rates of gambling were increasing. This included increases in the proportions of gamblers that had turned to online gambling. This behaviour characterised male more than female gamblers and was also predicted by having a high income, being unemployed and being a homemaker or retiree among other factors. Moving online was also linked to a greater volume of gambling and with problem gambling. In fact, the predictors indicated that the potential problems caused by online gambling could affect many different types of people. Although being male emerged as a significant predictor of online gambling, so too did being a homemaker, which was more likely to mean being a woman. People with more money to spend might indulge in gambling and so also would those without much money, quite possibly for different reasons (Pallesen et al., 2021).

A number of studies were carried out in different parts of the world to assess whether people's gambling habits did change during the pandemic compared with before it. The closure of many gambling outlets led to reductions in rates of gambling for a time in some countries. Research in New Zealand found that for around half of people who gambled that were questioned, they mentioned financial reasons for not gambling as much. Others did not want to be seen gambling around family members with whom they were ensconced at home.

In the United Kingdom, the closure of live sports events on which the gamble was the most frequent reason but other reasons mentioned by fewer included having less money to spend, loss of interest in gambling during the pandemic and a weakened inclination to spend of lotteries (Gunstone et al., 2020).

Other research indicated increased rates of gambling in some populations (Fluharty et al., 2020; Gainsbury et al., 2020; Gunstone et al., 2020; Health Promotion Agency, 2020). A few surveys revealed increased online gambling specifically (Abacus Data, 2020; Brown & Hickman, 2020; Gunstone et al., 2020; Jenkinson et al., 2020; Leonard et al., 2021; Health Promotion Agency, 2020; Xuereb et al., 2021). Looking across these studies, reported population-wide gambling increased by between 11% and 20%.

Swedish research compared early pandemic gambling levels with benchmark data for 2016 in a general population survey. There was an overall increase in gambling overall of 4% during the early part of the pandemic compared with four years earlier. This change occurred despite the cancellation of major sports events. Not everyone responded in the same way, of course. The proportions of people reporting an increase in their gambling behaviour outweighed the proportions reporting a decrease in respect of online casinos, online horse betting and online lotteries. In general, only a minority of gamblers said they had increased how much they gambled during the pandemic, but among those individuals, problem gamblers were over-represented (Håkansson, 2020a).

One review of 17 studies about gambling during the pandemic concluded that with the closure of many sports events and offline gambling venues, the overall volume of gambling declined during the pandemic when societies were locked down. Where gambling behaviour did increase, whether among problem gamblers or gamblers in general it was associated with being male and younger, and also often resulted in problematic gambling (Hodgins & Stevens, 2021; Shaw et al., 2021). In several instances, it was not just gambling in general that increased, but more seriously, rates of problem gambling increased (Gunstone et al., 2020; Håkansson, 2020; Xuereb et al., 2021). Increased gambling was found to occur among many sections of populations, but there was more evidence to show that reports of this behaviour were more prevalent among younger people (Abacus Data, 2020; Biddle, 2020; Brown & Hickman, 2020; Jenkinson et al., 2020; Health Promotion Agency, 2020). Men were found to be at risk of increased gambling (Biddle, 2020; Gunstone et al., 2020; Jenkinson et al., 2020) and evidence also emerged that women could be as well (Gainsbury et al., 2020). People who reported increased gambling were also more likely than others to report anxiety and depression symptoms, consumed more alcohol and were more likely to dabble with drugs (Bonny-Noach & Gold, 2020; Fluharty et al., 2020; Håkansson, 2020).

In a large-sample nationwide survey of people's behaviours during the pandemic, Fluharty et al. (2020) found that gambling during strict lockdown periods was predicted by a number of variables including being male, being in an older age bracket, being employed, having a lower level of education, living in overcrowded accommodation, being heavier consumers of alcohol and being bored. Signs of anxiety and depression also added to the mix in increasing risk of gambling during periods of tight behaviour restrictions (Fluharty et al., 2020).

As suggested above, even though having less money during the pandemic emerged as a reason for reduced gambling, other evidence emerged from some populations that gambling was seen as a means of fixing personal financial problems caused by pandemic-related job loss and reduction in income (Centre for the Advancement of Best Practices Responsible Gambling Council, 2020; Price, 2020; 38] Online gambling as also so convenient and gamblers could still play even though largely restricted to staying in their own homes (Price, 2020).

Problem Gambling and COVID-19

Carried to an extreme, or at least beyond what the individual can afford, gambling can cause harm to players and their families (Hodgins et al., 2011; Langham et al., 2016). It can display many of the qualities of an addiction. Problem gamblers keep gambling even when they keep losing at it. Gambling becomes a priority in their lives and other aspects of their lives get side-lined and suffer (Saunders, 2017). Some gamblers focus on one form of gambling, but many problem gamblers play many different formats (Allami et al., 2021).

The interventions deployed by many governments against the pandemic resulted in the closure of large parts of their economies. Many people suffered job losses or reduced incomes as a result. Turning to gambling as a means of gaining financial compensation for reduced incomes often mane players personal financial circumstances even worse (Campbell, 2020; van Schalkwyk et al., 2020). For some, restrictions on movements created repetitive daily routines devoid of normal social stimulation that were monotonous. Boredom often led to anxiety and this in turn encourage people to turn to distraction activities that remained available (Brooks et al., 2020; Asmundson & Taylor, 2020). Such psychological states were already known to create conditions that could encourage gambling and especially problem gambling (Mercer & Eastwood, 2010; Lorains et al., 2011).

Counterbalancing these effects, pandemic-related restrictions on sports could reduce the range of events available for gamblers to place bets on. Loss of income might encourage some people to resist spending the money they had left on high-risk pursuits (Olason et al., 2015; Olason et al., 2017). The impact of physical distancing measures however might encourage others to engage with gambling activities where this gave them the opportunity to join with gambling communities and to experience some sense of social substitution for the social deprivation conditions imposed upon them (Håkansson et al., 2017; Ramnerö et al., 2019).

Problem gambling has been linked to psychological problems such as stress and during the pandemic, this was widely experienced. It was also found to be linked to online gambling and live sports betting. It can arise from both offline and online gambling (Marmet et al., 2021). During the pandemic, much of the former was suspended as live sports events were banned. Online gambling, however, was widely available still and as the only gambling option that remained open to many gamblers, understandably attracted a lot of interest. Online gambling was also associated with borrowing money for and getting into debt over gambling, and this over-indebtedness was disproportionately likely to occur among online casino gamblers (Håkansson, & Widinghoff, 2020).

One study compared gambling levels before and after the pandemic had started rather than just during its initial phases. The researchers obtained data provided by a large European online gambling company with players spread across Germany, Norway, Sweden and Finland. Gambling data were analysed before and after 7th March 2020. The starting point for data collection was to gather data for all bettors that placed at least one bet in at least five weeks out of ten between 1st January and 7th March 2020. The results showed a decrease in online casino betting and little evidence of sports bettors switching across to casino betting. Sports betting wagers declined during the pandemic compared with before it and sports bettors did not switch to other forms of betting, at least within this one betting company (Auer et al., 2020).

Research conducted in Canada showed that a rise in online gambling during the pandemic was most likely to be seen in those classified as high-risk gamblers. These were people with prior experience of online gambling who had also often migrated across from land-based gambling. Further evidence indicated that problem gamblers also exhibited higher than average levels of anxiety, had reduced hours of work during the pandemic and perceived that they were being influenced to gamble by the events of the pandemic, and gambled under the influence of alcohol or cannabis. Some also suffered from depression and turned to gambling as a measure for alleviating adverse mental health symptoms such as being nervous and depressed (Price, 2020).

As a backdrop to these observations in Canada, the country had experienced falling employment rates and these continued during the pandemic. These trends had had a negative impact on the status of public mental health. It was therefore somewhat reassuring that overall levels of gambling did not increase during the pandemic. Increased gambling rates were, as elsewhere, largely confined to those already most at risk of problem gambling (see also, Håkansson, 2020b).

Yet, narratives about the risks of gambling continued to appear during the pandemic. There was a widespread belief that social isolation could aggravate specific mental health concerns and that these in turn could create the right psychological states for problem gambling to occur (Douglas et al., 2020; Marsden et al., 2020).

Pre-pandemic research reported links between problem gambling and mental health problems (LaPlante et al., 2008; Hing et al., 2016; Gainsbury, 2015; Awaworyi et al., 2018). In essence, those who developed a gambling problem not unusually also showed other mental health difficulties. Among the other problem behaviours were excess alcohol consumption and depression (Griffiths & Parke, 2010). Depression was also found to be linked to gambling in many different types of gambling game and to a preference in particular for casino betting and sports betting (McBride & Derevensky, 2009; Lloyd et al., 2010b).

Price (2020) found that gamblers who gambled regularly before the pandemic gambled less online than they had offline once the emergency measures had been instigated, but they still represented most of the online gamblers at this time. Gamblers who had reported playing a range of gambling games before the pandemic were among the heaviest online gamblers during it, at least during the first six weeks after emergency measures had started. Those classified as "non-problem" gamblers exhibited more modest rates of online gambling during the pandemic. High-risk gamblers before the pandemic were nine times as likely as low-risk gamblers to gamble during the pandemic.

Further evidence showed that other mental health problems were linked to the probabilities of pandemic gambling. Respondents with no symptoms of anxiety or depression were less likely to gamble than were those displaying these symptoms. Hence, gambling likelihood during the pandemic was increased when gamblers were anxious or depressed. The financial circumstances of respondents, that had often been affected by the pandemic, also showed a relationship to online gambling during the health crisis period. Gambling was more likely to be reported by respondents who reported losing their jobs or having had their hours of work reduced after the pandemic hit (Price, 2020).

The Pandemic and Use of Gambling Support Services

Concerns that the pandemic would drive an increase in gambling were also linked to fears that there would be an increased demand for support for problem gamblers that might not be available in the usual formats as public health services directed more of their resources towards coping with the pandemic and with face-to-face consultations being largely suspended (Sveriges Television [Swedish Television] (2020a, 2020b). Moreover, many problem gamblers might be reluctant to seek help under the extreme circumstances created by the pandemic (Håkansson et al., 2020).

Another method of assessing when the pandemic had influenced gambling behaviour was to investigate the activity at gambling disorder centres set up to support people for whom their gambling had got out of control. One such study in Sweden compared 2020 pandemic levels of use month by month with data for similar periods in 2018 and 2019. The data did not show any increase in treatment uptake for gambling problems during the early months after COVID-19 had been detected in Sweden as compared with pre-pandemic periods (Hakansson et al., 2021).

As this analysis covered the first 10 months of the pandemic, the researchers cautioned that further research might be needed over a longer time period to be sure there were no lasting effects of the pandemic on the behaviour of problem gamblers. Because the study focused on a highly specialist support unit, this restricted the size and composition of the sample which could also have affected the results. Even so, on a limited scale, there was some indicative evidence of an increase in the use of this support centre, even though not in the form of seeking direct treatment on the support unit's premises. While not being robust enough to confirm a pandemic effect, the findings invited further data collection of this kind.

Other factors were known to come into play in relation to the use of these support centres. Some problem gamblers were known to be fearful about using this kind of support. This resistance has been found for the use of health support systems for other kinds of addiction (Columb et al., 2020; Glowacki et al., 2021; Mellis et al., 2021). The Swedish clinic under investigation found that many of its contacts preferred to speak over the telephone or via video links rather than in person at the facility. Distance treatment services are therefore important to reach out to people in need of help but too anxious to turn up physically to help facilities.

Overview of Gambling and the Pandemic

As their lives were put on hold by the pandemic and accompanying government restrictions, many people turned to those pursuits that remained available to them. Among these was gambling. For established gamblers, the closure of most major sports competitions meant that these disappeared as their usual betting options. There were the usual concerns voiced about the dangers of more people becoming hooked on gambling and betting beyond their means. At the same time, betting firms and even the World Health Organization endorsed gambling, within reason, as a good way to alleviate the boredom of pandemic lockdowns.

One critical question was whether there was hard evidence that the boredom and anxiety caused to many by being asked to stay home and rarely venture out and to avoid seeing people, including close relatives, from different households, would motivate more people to gambling more than they should. In answering this question, it is essential to know how much people actually did gamble when they went online. Such evidence as did emerge during the pandemic was equivocal on this point. There were some data that indicated an increased interest in online gambling. This was manifest in longer gambling sessions rather than more of them. There was also some indication that for some types of betting, gambling revenues increased during the pandemic compared with pre-pandemic comparison periods.

Some types of online gambling, linked to sports events, disappeared as those events were closed down. Gamblers accustomed to betting on these events did shift to other forms of gambling. Online lotteries, online casino games and online slots gambling showed increased use in some markets. This behaviour was dominated by established and problem gamblers.

Increased gambling during the pandemic was not unexpected. Similar behaviour had been observed during previous crises, such as the 2008 financial markets crash. There was therefore a genuine worry that the restrictions on everyday activities during the 2020 coronavirus outbreak would give more people more time to fill. The closure of most of society also meant that for many people still in active employment, their opportunities to spend money on leisure and entertainment were also restricted. This might have set the scene for gambling to be taken up by former non-gamblers. Instead, any increased gambling activity was largely restricted to established and problem gamblers. Among these individuals, some switching around in their gambling pursuits was also noted at this time. As sports betting disappeared with sports events, gamblers often switched to online casino games. Among the new online gamblers, most were already established offline gamblers that still needed a gambling fix.

In terms of potential psychological damage, it was already known that mental health problems had been linked to excess gambling even before the pandemic. The pandemic itself created conditions in which those prone to develop psychological problems became more prone to do so. Combining pandemic anxiety and gambling stress among those losing more than they should, could have presented a dangerous cocktail of conditions for those prone to develop mental health problems. Despite this concern, no evidence emerged of significant increases in the use of gambling support services. If gambling had contributed to increased prevalence of mental health problems during the coronavirus pandemic, therefore, it was not evidenced in the volume of problem gamblers seeking help.

Overall then the picture for the impact of the pandemic on gambling is mixed. Reduced opportunities to gamble, caused by the closure of all sports events, drove forcibly drove down many popular types of gambling. For some gamblers, this meant suspension of their usual gambling activities. For others, compensatory activities were sought out online. These were readily available and even more extensively so than were traditional land-based forms of gambling. Any shift to online gambling was regarded by gambling regulators as problematic because of the ease with which it enabled habitual gamblers to satisfy their urges to gamble. This form of gambling was known to be linked to onset of problem gambling and for the most serious players high levels of gambling losses that many could not afford. Moreover, many online gambling games originated outside the countries in which they were played and therefore could not be controlled by local regulatory codes and laws.

References

Abacus Data. (2020). Online gambling/betting: a survey of 1,500 Canadians during the COVID-19 pandemic. Toronto, Canada. Retrieved from: https://www.greo.ca/Modules/EvidenceCentre/Details/online-gambling-betting-a-survey-of-1–500-canadians-during-the-covid-19-pandemic

Abel, T. & McQueen, D. (2020). The COVID-19 pandemic calls for spatial distancing and social closeness: Not for social distancing! *International Journal of Public Health*, 65(3): 231. https://doi.org/10.1007/s00038-020-01366-7

Addiction Policy Forum. (2020). Free smartphone app offering telehealth support for those struggling with addiction during COVID-19. Retrieved from: https://www.addictionpolicy.org/post/free-smartphone-app-offering-telehealth-support-for-those-struggling-with-addiction-during-covid-19

Allami, Y., Hodgins, D. C., Young, M., et al. (2021). A meta-analysis of problem gambling risk factors in the general adult population. *Addiction*, 16(11): 2968–2977. doi: 10.1111/add.15449

Asmundson, G. J. G. & Taylor, S. (2020). How health anxiety influences responses to viral outbreaks like COVID-19: what all decision-makers, health authorities, and health care professionals need to know. *Journal of Anxiety Disorders*, 71: 102211. doi: 10.1016/j.janxdis.2020.102211

Auer, M. Malischnig, D., & Griffiths, M. (2020). Gambling before and during the COVID-19 pandemic among european regular sports bettors: An empirical study using behavioral tracking data. *International Journal of Mental Health and Addiction*, 1–8. Retrieved from: 10.1007/s11469-020-00327-8

Awaworyi Churchill, S. & Farrell, L. (2018). The impact of gambling on depression: New evidence from England and Scotland. *Economic Modelling*, 68(C): 475–483.

Biddle, N. (2020). Gambling during the COVID-19 pandemic: ANU Centre for Social Research and Methods and Centre for Gambling Research. Retrieved from: https://csrm.cass.anu.edu.au/sites/default/files/docs/2020/12/Gambling_during_the_COVID-19_pandemic.pdf

Billieux, J., Flayelle, M., Rumpf, H. J., & Stein, D. J. (2019). High involvement versus pathological involvement in video games: A crucial distinction for ensuring the validity and utility of gaming disorder. *Current Addiction Reports*, 6: 323–330.

Binde, P., Romild, U., & Volberg, R. A. (2017). Forms of gambling, gambling involvement and problem gambling: evidence from a Swedish population survey. *International Gambling Studies*, 17: 490–507. doi: 10.1080/14459795.2017.1360928

Bonny-Noach, H., & Gold, D. (2020). Addictive behaviors and craving during the COVID-19 pandemic of people who have recovered from substance use disorder. *Journal of Addictive Disease*, 39: 1–20.

Brooks, S. K., Webster, R. K., Smith, L. E., Woodland, L., Wessely, S., Greenberg, N., et al. (2020). The psychological impact of quarantine and how to reduce it: Rapid review of the evidence. *Lancet*, 395: 912–920. doi: 10.1016/S0140-6736(20) 30460-8

Brown, R., & Hickman, A. (2020, June). *Changes in online gambling during the COVID-19 pandemic: Statistical Bulletin 25*, April Update. Australian Institute of Criminology, Analysis & Policy Observatory. Retrieved from: https://apo.org. au/node/306090

Businesswire. (2020). Games industry unites to promote World Health Organization messages against COVID-19; Launch #PlayApartTogether campaign. Retrieved March 31, 2020, from: https://www.businesswire.com/news/home/ 20200328005018/en/Games-Industry-Unites-Promote-World-Health-Organization

Campbell, C. (2020). Coronavirus: Lockdown leaves addicts 'close to relapse'. *BBC News*, 27 May 2020. https://www.bbc.com/news/uk-northern-ireland-52811931 [Accessed 28 January2021]

Carras, M. C., Van Rooij, A. J., Van de Mheen, D., Musci, R., Xue, Q. L., & Mendelson, T. (2017). Video gaming in a hyperconnected world: A cross-sectional study of heavy gaming, problematic gaming symptoms, and online socializing in adolescents. *Computers in Human Behavior*, 68: 472–479.

Centre for the Advancement of Best Practices Responsible Gambling Council. (2020). *The Emerging Impact of COVID-19 on Gambling in Ontario*. Toronto, Ontario: Author.

Columb, D., Hussain, R., & O'Gara, C. (2020). Addiction psychiatry and COVID-19: Impact on patients and service provision. *Irish Journal of Psychological Medicine*, 37: 164–168.

Corbin, W. R., Farmer, N. M., & Nolen-Hoekesma, S. (2013). Relations among stress, coping strategies, coping motives, alcohol consumption and related problems: A mediated moderation model. *Addictive Behaviors*, 38(4): 1912–1919.

Douglas, M., Kalikireddi, S. V., Taulbut, M., McKee, M., & McCartney, G. (2020). Mitigating the wider health effects ofcovid-19 pandemic: response. The BMJ, 369: m1557. Retrieved from: https://www.bmj.com/content/bmj/369/bmj.m1557.full.pdf

Financial Times. (2020). Gamblers Bet on Marbles and Trotting as Pandemic Hits Sport. Financial Times. 2020. Available online: https://www.ft.com/content/ 71aa11ad-cf3e-47b3–8cfe-9233c436ea32 (accessed on 10 December 2020).

Fluharty, M., Paul, E., & Fancourt, D. (2020). Predictors and patterns of gambling behaviour across the COVID-19 lockdown: findings from a UK cohort study 10.31234/osf.io/8qthw

Gainsbury, S. M. (2015). Online gambling addiction: the relationship between Internet gambling and disordered gambling. *Current Addiction* Reports, 2: 185–193.

Gainsbury, S. M., Swanton, T. B., Burgess, M. T., & Blaszczynski, A. (2020). Impacts of the COVID-19 shutdown on gambling patterns in Australia: consideration of problem gambling and psychological distress. *Journal of Addictive Medicine*, Publish Ahead of Print. doi: 10.1097/ADM.0000000000000793

Ghebreyesus, T. A. (2020). Thank you @RaymondChambers for mobilizing the gaming industry to feature @WHO advice on #COVID19 to their users. We must all #PlayApartTogether to beat the #coronavirus. 9:29 am. 29 March 2020. Tweet. Geneva, Switzerland: World Health Organization.

Glowacki, E. M., Wilcox, G. B., & Glowacki, J. B. (2021). Identifying #addiction concerns on twitter during the COVID-19 pandemic: A text mining analysis. *Substance Abuse*, 42: 39–46.

Granic, I., Lobel, A., & Engels, R. C. (2014). The benefits of playing video games. *American Psychologist*, 69(1): 66–78.

Griffiths, M. D. (20110 Adolescent gambling. In B. Bradford-Brown & M. Prinstein (Eds.) *Encyclopaedia of Adolescence*, Vol. 3, pp. 11–20. San Diego, CA: Academic Press. doi:10.1016/B978-0-12-373915-5.00113-3

Griffiths, M. D., & Parke, J. (2010). Adolescent gambling on the internet: a review. *International Journal of Adolescent Medicine & Health*, 22(1): 59–75.

Gunstone, B., Gosschalk, K., Joyner, O., Diaconu, A., & Sheikh, M. (2020). The impact of the COVID19 lockdown on gambling behaviour, harms and demand for treatment and support. London. https://about.gambleaware.org/media/2284/yougov-covid-19-report.pdf.

Håkansson, A. (2020a). Changes in gambling behavior during the COVID-19 pandemic – A web survey study in Sweden. *International Journal of Environmental Research and Public Health*, 17: 4013.

Håkansson, A. (2020b). Impact of COVID-19 on online gambling – a general population survey during the pandemic. *Frontiers in Psychology*, 11: 568543.

Håkansson, A. (2020c). Changes in gambling behavior during the COVID-19 pandemic: A web survey study in Sweden. *International Journal of Environmental Research and Public Health*, 17(4013): 1–16. 10.3390/ijerph17114013

Hakansson, A., Akesson, G., Grudet, C., & Broman, N. (2021). No apparent increase in treatment uptake for gambling disorder during ten months of the COVUD-19 pandemic – analysis of a regional specialized treatment unit in Sweden. *International Journal of Environmental Research and Public Health*, 18(4): 1918. doi: 10.2290.ijerph18041918

Håkansson, A., Fernández-Aranda, F., Menchón, J. M., Potenza, M. N., & Jiménez-Murcia, S. (2020). Gambling during the COVID-19 crisis—A cause for concern. *Journal of Addiction and Medicine*, 14(4): e10–e12.

Håkansson, A., Mårdhed, E., & Zaar M. (2017). Who seeks treatment when medicine opens the door to pathological gambling patients – psychiatric comorbidity and heavy predominance of online gambling. *Frontiers of Psychiatry*, 8: 6–11. doi: 10.3389/fpsyt.2017.00255

Håkansson, A. & Widinghoff, C. (2020). Over-indebtedness and problem gambling in a general population sample of online gamblers. *Frontiers in Psychiatry*, 11: 7. doi: 10.3389/fpsyt.2020.00007

Health Promotion Agency. (2020). *The impact of lockdown on health risk behaviours* Wellington, New Zealand. Retrieved from: https://www.hpa.org.nz/research-library/research-publications/the-impact-of-lockdown-on-health-risk-behaviours

Hing, N., Russell, A. M. T., Vitartas, P. *et al.* (2016). Demographic, Behavioural and Normative Risk Factors for Gambling Problems Amongst Sports Bettors. *Journal of Gambling Studies*, 32(625–641): 2016. 10.1007/s10899-015-9571-9

Hodgins, D. C., Stea, J. N., & Grant, J. E. (2011). Gambling disorders. *Lancet*, 378: 1874–1884.

Hodgins, D. C. & Stevens, R. M. G. (2021). The Impact of COVID-19 on gambling and gambling disorder: emerging data. *Current Opinion in Psychiatry*, 34(4): 332–343.

Holmes, E. A., O'Connor, R. C.,Perry, V. H., Tracey, I., Wessely, S., Arseneault, L., Ballard, C., Christensen, H., Silver, R. C., Everall, I., et al. (2020). Multidisciplinary research priorities for the COVID-19 pandemic: A call for action for mental health science. *Lancet Psychiatry*, 7: 547–560.

Horner, A. (2020). Online casinos searchers a 'all-time high' during lockdown. *BBC News*. Retrieved from: https://www.bbc.com/news/uk-england-52633355

Javed, J. (2020). eSports and gaming industry thriving as video games provide escape from reality during coronavirus pandemic. Retrieved from: https://www.wfaa.com/article/sports/esports-gaming-industry-thriving-as-video-games-provide-escape-from-reality-during-coronavirus-pandemic/287-5953d982-d240-4e2b-a2ba-94dd60a8a383

Jenkinson, R., Sakata, K., Khokhar, T., et al. (2020). Gambling in Australia during COVID-19. Southbank, Victoria, Australia, https://www.greo.ca/Modules/EvidenceCentre/Details/gambling-in-australia-during-covid19

King, D. L.Gaming Industry Response Consortium (2018). Comment on the global gaming industry's statement on ICD-11 gaming disorder: A corporate strategy to disregard harm and deflect social responsibility? *Addiction*, 113: 2145–2146.

King, D. L. & Delfabbro, P. H. (2020). Problematic online gaming and the COVID-19 pandemic. *Journal of Behavioural Addictions*, 9(2): 184–186.

King, D. L., Delfabbro, P. H., Billieux, J., & Potenza, M. N. (2020). Problematic online gaming and the COVID-19 pandemic. *Journal of Behavioural Addictictions*, 9: 184–186.

King, D., Koster, E., & Billieux, J. (2019). Study what makes games addictive. *Nature*, 573: 346–346.

Király, O., Tóth, D., Urbán, R., Demetrovics, Z., & Maraz, A. (2017). Intense video gaming is not essentially problematic. *Psychology of Addictive Behaviors*, 31: 807–817.

Langham, E., Thorne, H., Browne, M., et al. (2016). Understanding gambling related harm: A proposed definition, conceptual framework, and taxonomy of harms. *BMC Public Health*, 16: 80.

LaPlante, D. A., Schumann, A., LaBrie, R. A., & Shaffer, H. J. (2008). Population trends in Internet sports gambling. *Computers in Human Behavior*, 24(5): 2399–2414.

Leonard, C. A., Williams, R. J., & McGrath, D. S. (2021). Gambling fallacies: Predicting problem gambling in a national sample. *Psychology of Addictive Behaviors*, 35(8): 939–947. https://doi.org/10.1037/adb0000673

Lepido, D. & Rolander, N. (2020). Housebound Italian kids strain network with Fortnite marathon. Retrieved from: https://www.bloomberg.com/news/articles/2020-03-12/housebound-italian-kids-strain-network-with-fortnite-marathon

Lindner, P., Forsström, D., Jonsson, J., Berman, A. H., & Carlbring, P. (2020). Transitioning between online gambling modalities and decrease in total gambling activity, but no indication of increases in problematic online gambling intensity during the first phase of the COVID-19 outbreak in Sweden: A time series forecast study. *Frontiers in Public Health*, 8: 554542.

Lischer, S., Steffen, A., Schwarz, J., & Mathys, J. (2021). The influence of lockdown on the gambling pattern of Swiss casino players. *International Journal of Environmental Research and Public Health*, 18(4): 1073. Doi: 10.3390/ijerph18041973

Lloyd, J., Doll, H., Hawton, K., Dutton, W. H., Geddes, J. R., Goodwin, G. M., & Rogers, R. D. (2010a). Internet gamblers: A latent class analysis of their behaviours and health experiences. *Journal of Gambling Studies*, 26(3): 387–399. doi: 10.1007/s10899-010-9188-y

Lloyd, J., Doll, H., Hawton, K., Dutton, W. H., Geddes, J. R., Goodwin, G. M., & Rogers, R. D. (2010b). How psychological symptoms relate to different motivations for gambling: An online study of internet gamblers. *Biological Psychiatry*, 68(8): 733–740. doi: 10.1016/j.biopsych.2010.03.038

Lorains, F. K., Cowlishaw, S., & Thomas, S. A. (2011). Prevalence of comorbid disorders in problem and pathological gambling: Systematic review and meta-analysis of population surveys. *Addiction*, 106: 490–498. doi: 10.1111/j.1360-0443.2010.03300.x

Maden, A. (2020). World Health Organization encourages people to game during coronavirus outbreak. Retrieved March 31, 2020, from: https://www.windowscentral.com/world-health-organization-encourages-people-game-during-coronavirus-outbreak

Marmet, S., Studer, J., Wicki, M., Khazaal, Y., & Gmel G. (2021). Online gambling's associations with gambling disorder and related problems in a representative sample of young Swiss men. *Frontiers of Psychiatry*, 12: 703118. doi: 10.3389/fpsyt.2021.703118

Marsden, J., Darke, S., Hall, W., Hickman, M., Holmes, J., Humphreys, K., Neale, J., Tucker, J., & West, R. (2020). Mitigating and learning from the impact of COVID-19 infection on addictive disorders. *Addiction*, 115(6): 1007–1010. doi: 10.1111/add.15080

McBride, J. & Derevensky, J. (2009). Internet gambling behaviour in a sample of online gamblers. *International Journal of Mental Health and Addiction*, 7(1): 149–167. 10.1007/s11469-008-9169-x

Mellis, A. M., Potenza, M. N., & Hulsey, J. N. (2021). COVID-19-related treatment service disruptions among people with single- and polysubstance use concerns. *Journal of Substance Abuse and Treatment*, 121: 108180.

Mercer, K. B., & Eastwood, J. D. (2010). Is boredom associated with problem gambling behaviour? It depends on what you mean by 'boredom'. *International Gambling Studies*, 10: 91–104. doi: 10.1080/14459791003754414

Olason, D. T., Hayer, T., Brosowski, T., & Meyer G. (2015). Gambling in the mist of economic crisis: Results from three national prevalence studies from Iceland. *Journal of Gambling Studies*, 31: 759–774. doi: 10.1007/s10899-015-9523-4

Olason, D. T., Hayer, T., Meyer, G., & Brosowski, T. (2017). Economic recession affects gambling participation but not problematic gambling: Results from a population-based follow-up study. *Frontiers of Psychology*, 8: 1247. doi: 10.3389/fpsyg.2017.01247

Pallesen, S., Mentzoni, R. A., Morken, A. M., Engebø, J., Kaur, P., & Erevik, E. K. (2021). Changes over time and predictors of online gambling in three Norwegian population studies 2013-2019. *Frontiers of Psychiatry*, 12: 597615. doi: 10.3389/fpsyt.2021.597615

Pantling, A. (2020). Gaming usage up 75 percent amid coronavirus outbreak, Verizon reports. Retrieved from: https://www.hollywoodreporter.com/news/gaming-usage-up-75-percent-coronavirus-outbreak-verizon-reports-1285140

Perez, M. (2020). Video games are being played at record levels as the coronavirus keeps people indoors. Retrieved from: https://www.forbes.com/sites/mattperez/2020/03/16/video-games-are-being-played-at-record-levels-as-the-coronavirus-keeps-people-indoors/#70eb644e57ba

Potenza, M. N., Balodis, I. M., Derevensky, J., Grant, J. E., Petry, N. M., Verdejo-Garcia, A., & Yip, S. W. (2019). Gambling disorder. *National Reviews Disease Primers*, 5: 51. doi: 10.1038/s41572-019-0099-7

Price, A. (2020). Online gambling in the *midst* of COVID-19: A nexus of mental health concerns, substance use and financial stress. *International Journal of Mental Health and Addiction*, 1–18. Retrieved from: 10.1007/s11469-020-00366-1

Ramnerö, J., Molander, O., Lindner, P., & Carlbring P. (2019). What can be learned about gambling from a learning perspective? A narrative review. *Nordic Psychology*, 71: 303–322. doi: 10.1080/19012276.2019.1616320

Razzoli, M., Pearson, C., Crow, S., & Bartolomucci, A. (2017). Stress, overeating, and obesity: Insights from human studies and preclinical models. *Neuroscience & Biobehavioral Reviews*, 76: 154–162.

Reuters, (2020). Sweden to Limit Online Betting during Coronavirus Outbreak. Reuters. 2020. Available online: https://www.reuters.com/article/us-health-coronavirus-sweden-gambling/sweden-to-limit-online-betting-during-coronavirusoutbreak-idUSKCN2251WC (accessed on 10 December 2020).

Saunders, J. B. (2017). Substance use and addictive disorders in DSM-5 and ICD 10 and the draft ICD 11. *Current Opinion in Psychiatry*, 30: 227–237.

Saunders, J. B., Hao, W., Long, J., King, D. L., Mann, K., & Fauth-Bühler, M., (2017). Gaming disorder: Its delineation as an important condition for diagnosis, management, and prevention. *Journal of Behavioral Addictions*, 6: 271–279.

S. B. C. News. (2020). Spain Order 'Social Shield' to Fast Track Gambling Advertising Window. SBC News. 2020. Available online: https://sbcnews.co.uk/europe/2020/04/01/spain-orders-social-shield-to-fast-track-gambling-advertising-window/ (accessed on 10December2020).

Shaw, C. A., Hodgins, D. C., Williams, R. J., Belanger, Y. D., Christensen, D. R., El-Guebaly, N., McGrath, D. S., Nicoll, F., Smith, G. J., & Stevens, R. (2021). Gambling in Canada During the COVID Lockdown: Prospective National Survey. *Journal of gambling studies*, 1–26. . 10.1007/s10899-021-10073-8

Stephen, B. (2020). This is Twitch's moment [internet]. Retrieved from: https://www.theverge.com/2020/3/18/21185114/twitch-youtube-livestreaming-streamelements-coronavirus-quarantine-viewership-numbers

Sveriges Television [Swedish Television] (2020a). *Fler Söker Stöd för Spelberoende Under Coronapandemin.* [More People Seek Support for Gambling Problems during the Corona Pandemic]. Available online: https://www.svt.se/nyheter/lokalt/skane/fler-sokerstod-for-spelberoende-under-coronapandemin (accessed on 10 December 2020).

Sveriges Television [Swedish Television].(2020b) *Kraftig Ökning av Spelberoende Som Söker Hjälp.* [Large Increase in Number of Individuals Addicted to Gambling Who Seek Help]. Available online: https://www.svt.se/nyheter/lokalt/vast/paskhelg-ochcoronapandemi-farlig-tid-for-spelberoende (accessed on 10 December 2020).

The Gambling Commission (2021, 20th January). Data shows the impact of COVID-19 on gambling behaviour in November 2020. Retrieved from: https://www.gamblingcommission.gov.uk/news-action-and-statistics/news/2021/Data-shows-the-impact-of-Covid-19-on-gambling-behaviour-in-November-2020.aspx

The Guardian (2020). Coronavirus: Gambling firms urged to impose betting cap of L50 a day. *The Guardian*. Available online: https://www.theguardian.com/sport/2020/mar/22/coronavirus-gambling-firms-urged-to-impose-betting-cap-of-50-a-day (accessed on 10 December 2020).

Torales, J., O'Higgins, M., Castaldelli-Maia, J. M., & Ventriglio, A. (2020). The outbreak of COVID-19 coronavirus and its impact on global mental health. *International Journal of Social Psychiatry*, 66(4): 317–320. doi: 10.1177/0020764020915212.

van Schalkwyk, M. C. I., Heetham, D., Reeves, A., & Petticrew, M. (2020). We must take urgent action to avoid an increase in problem gambling and gambling related harms. *The BMJ*, https://blogs.bmj.com/bmj/2020/04/06/covid-19-we-must-take-urgent-action-to-avoid-an-increase-in-problem-gambling-and-gambling-related-harms/

Wells, I. (2020, 29th April). Coronavirus pandemic 'a disaster' for gambling addicts. *BBC News*. Retrieved from: https://www.bbc.co.uk/news/uk-wales-politics-52460269

Wood, R. T., & Williams, R. J. (2011). A comparative profile of the Internet gambler: Demographic characteristics, game-play patterns, and problem gambling status. *New Media and Society*, 13: 1123–1141.

World Health Organization. (2020). #HealthyAtHome – Mental Health. Retrieved from: https://www.who.int/news-room/campaigns/connecting-the-world-to-combat-coronavirus/healthyathome/healthyathome---mental-health

Xuereb, S., Kim, H. S., Clark, L., & Wohl, M. J. A. (2021). Substitution behaviors among casino gamblers during COVID-19 precipitated casino closures. *International Gambling Studies*. [E-publication ahead of print] 10.1080/14459795.2021.1903062

Chapter 11

Re-Setting Public Behaviour

Evidence from an analysis of early pandemic news stories and research across the first two years of the pandemic indicated that there was a lot of attention given to rising anxiety and depression levels because of the stress of being locked down (Kim, 2020; Brunier & Drysdale, 2022). There was a lot of negative rhetoric in circulation during the first month of the initial United Kingdom lockdown. Stories also focused on other negative outcomes of lockdown such as increased domestic violence and marital breakdowns. Yet, lockdown also gave people time to reflect on their lives, evaluate what was really important to them and to re-set their lives.

There were many potential positives to take from this extreme event, but this was not the focus of much of the news coverage. Most of all, the news concentrated on infection levels and hospitalisation and death rates. There was no doubt, as evidence examined from elsewhere in this volume has indicated, that many people did experience negative emotions during the pandemic. At the same time, it also presented opportunities to recognise what was important in life, to connect better with family members and to appreciate that gratification could be obtained from simple things in life (Symonds, 2020).

Talk of a "new normal" during the pandemic has led many people to make adjustments to their lives involving behaviour changes that could be both positive and negative in their health outcomes. For example, there was evidence that the pandemic and the worry it caused was linked to increased alcohol consumption among some people, but decreased consumption among others. There was further evidence that some people had taken the new freedoms opened up by working from home or being laid off work temporarily to take more exercise. The choices that people make in terms of whether to be healthier or less healthy in their behaviour is linked to how anxious or depressed they get (Conroy & Nicholls, 2020). For those who managed to keep pandemic-related life changes in perspective or to perceive them as an opportunity to reset their lives, adopt more positive coping activities (Stevenson et al., 2019).

General compliance with pandemic restrictions was reported by the vast majority of people (96%) in the spring of 2021 (Fancourt et al., 2021).

DOI: 10.4324/9781003274377-11

As the pandemic wore on and with steadily growing numbers of people getting vaccinated in 2021, anxiety and depression levels by the spring of that year had stabilised and were similar to what they had been in May 2020. At this point in 2021, people's reports of their life satisfaction improved, returning to the level previously seen in summer 2020 when society had initially, temporarily opened up between lockdowns (Fancourt et al., 2021).

Lasting Effects: Mental Health

For many people, the pandemic will be remembered for the draconian restrictions placed on their everyday behaviours by their government. At some point, nearly all countries deployed a range of restrictive practices that were designed to minimise social and physical contact between people. This was regarded as the best way to bring a rapidly spreading, highly infectious and largely airborne disease under control. At their most extreme, these measures took the form of lockdown which was the closure of many of society's physical spaces where people interacted. This meant the closure of many workplaces, schools, universities, hospitality venues, sites of cultural, entertainment, leisure and sports activities and events and other locations. Entire publics were advised to stay home and to limit their trips outside to essential activities such as shopping for food, medicines and personal hygiene products or exercise for themselves and pets.

There was initial concern among many about catching the virus. Medical experts told everyone that most people suffered only mild symptoms at worst or none at all. Minorities would become unwell after being infected but only small minorities would need hospital treatment. The risks of needing intensive care were greatest among the oldest. While the last great pandemic – the Spanish flu outbreak of 1918 – affected young people more than older, the opposite was true of COVID-19 (Shanks & Brundage, 2012).

One of the greatest areas of concern about the lasting effects of COVID-19 was the impacts it had had on people's mental health. Anxiety levels rose and were widespread. They were triggered by worries about getting the virus, worries about losing jobs, the stresses of being confined to home most of the time and the deprivation experienced because of social isolation rules. Those working in frontline emergency and essential services, especially in healthcare and social care, also experienced huge stresses associated with much increased workloads that were relentless and also having to work in settings where their personal risks of infection increased.

Three out of four adults across the United Kingdom said they felt that their mental health was good or very good (77%) between April 2020 shortly after the first national lockdown had begun through to six months later in October 2020 before the second lockdown. More than one in seven (16%) reported that their mental health had declined during the early part of this period but then many reported that it improved again by the autumn

2020. The individuals that seemed to suffer the most without any obvious improvement in their condition were those with pre-existing physical and mental health problems (Pierce et al., 2021).

Fancourt and her colleagues conducted regular surveys with a panel of 70,000+ throughout the pandemic. In their 32nd set of results, there were findings concerning respondents' self-assessed mental health. Data released in March 2021 indicated a downturn in the proportion of people expressing feeling stressed about becoming seriously ill from COVID-19 (29%). Just over one in three people aged 18–59 years (34%) said they remained concerned about their finances by spring 2021 (Fancourt et al., 2021).

While general indicators showed that mental health status across the population as a whole remained fairly stable across the pandemic, there were notable variances among different population sub-groups. The prevalence of reported anxiety, stress and depression symptoms waxed and waned with lockdown implementation and release, but some parts of the populace suffered more than others and consistently reported more profound and adverse psychological reactions. Overall, women reported negative reactions more so than did men, young people (under 34) were more likely to report adverse symptoms than older people, and those with pre-existing mental or physical health symptoms also seemed to have a worse psychological journey through the pandemic than did most others.

Other mediating factors that magnified negative responses included membership of some ethnic minority groups, loss of employment and income and living in deprived neighbourhoods. It also became apparent that pre-existing psychological states could make a difference in how well people coped with the stresses caused by the pandemic. Individuals who generally felt they had less control over their lives and those who felt anxious about death were not as well equipped as most to cope with the impact of the pandemic and lockdown restrictions (Fancourt et al., 2020; Shevlin et al., 2020).

Lasting Effects of the Pandemic Experience for Children

School closures meant that extra pressures were placed on students and their families because of worries about being able to prepare properly for forthcoming exams and concerns about their longer-term futures. There were also the immediate stresses of families being at home together throughout the day, living on top of one another, as schoolchildren tried to adapt to studying at home and many parents adapted to working at home while also taking on roles as substitute teachers for their children.

Unsurprisingly there were early warnings about the impact of these scenarios on everyone's health and well-being (Bahn, 2020; Fegert et al., 2020; Holmes et al., 2020; Liu et al., 2020; Wang et al., 2020). Lockdown measures did not last forever, but they were re-instigated at least once in many countries as new waves of fresh variants of the coronavirus circulated. In coming out of the restrictions altogether, questions were then raised about what were the most serious psychological issues that confronted particular countries and their populations. Some of these problems were shared between countries and others were dependent on the nature of the restrictions imposed by governments and their timings.

With children, there were concerns about the impact of experience a pandemic had on their psychological state, about how this experience played out in their families and about the impact of schools being closed (Mental Health Foundation, 2021). The longer-term effects of the COVID-19 pandemic remain unknown at the time of writing this book. Lessons can be learned from research into the psychological effects of earlier pandemics. Of course, more recent or relatively recent pandemics (that is, which occurred in the 20th and 21st centuries) did not occur on the same scale as COVID-19, with the exception of the Spanish flu outbreak one hundred years earlier. Even so, local populations were often severely affected by these disease outbreaks and local authorities utilised different non-pharmaceutical measures to bring these epidemics and pandemics under control.

One of the key intervention measures deployed in pandemics is the quarantining of those infected. The experience of earlier pandemics, where relevant research was conducted, was that quarantine did not invariably produce lasting and serious psychological effects in those who had been quarantined during the H1N1 pandemic, compared with others that had not (Wang et al., 2011). In another investigation, conducted during the severe acute respiratory syndrome (SARS) epidemic in China, parents of quarantined children reported significantly higher rates of post-traumatic stress disorder compared to children that had not been quarantined (Sprang & Silman, 2013). Further studies confirmed that being quarantined could leave young people – children and adults – at increased risk of a range of mental health problems including chronic anxiety and stress and depression (Brooks et al., 2020; Liang et al., 2020; Saurabk & Ranjan, 2020; Xie et al., 2020).

Some young people had caring responsibilities for older relatives. These individuals were especially likely to report feeling the mental strain during the pandemic. They were expected to give emotional support but they did not always receive any when they needed it (Carers Trust, 2020). Likewise, healthcare workers reported stress symptoms because of the nature of their work. Many of these health professionals who were on the frontline could not also escape from the stressful impacts of lockdown within their own families (Brooks et al., 2020; Vindegaard & Benros, 2020).

There are a multitude of factors at play that contribute to stress and anxiety when people are quarantined. These included a fear of infection, loss of income and future financial uncertainty, worrying about other family members, shortages of supplies of essential commodities, social deprivation and loneliness and general frustration and boredom (see

Leigh-Hunt et al., 2017). Offsetting the longer-term impact of these variables will not be resolved through one action.

Extended and repeated closures of many schools for most pupils produced significant disruption to children's lives. Some tuition continued remotely but for many pupils, especially those from households with sparser technological resources, limited workspace and parents ill-equipped to provide home tuition support, their education was severely disrupted. Debates raged about the longer-term implications of this disruption on children's career prospects and quality of life. Children reported missing the academic and social aspects of school. There were concerns that their education had been disrupted with permanent repercussions (Mental Health Foundation 2020; Youth Link Scotland (2020). These concerns became especially acute for children who also had carer responsibilities at home (Carers Trust, 2020).

Despite the expectation that parents would share tuition duties with schoolteachers, in many households this did not happen all the time or at all. There was general concern among teachers that some pupils and their parents had failed to engage with the remote learning arrangements (Lucas et al., 2020). What this meant was the alternative model of learning that had to be applied almost by default for many households (exceptions being the children of parents who were essential workers and who continued to go into school). Hence, the longer-term educational implications of lockdown and school closures varied between pupils. Some would need greater assistance than others to catch up on lessons lost to COVID-19 (Lucas et al., 2020).

There were also variances in the degree of preparedness of schools for lockdown and the provision of remote tuition. One factor at play in this context was the sense of partnership between schools, local authorities and central government. This sense was often missing or only weakly formed (Waite et al., 2020). Such trust was also important going forward post-pandemic. All stakeholders needed to be ready to resume normal service and have in place effective strategies to enable children left behind during lockdown to catch up. Parents needed to have confidence that schools were able to provide such an effective educational environment and one that was safe, from a health standpoint, for their children to return to (Mental Health Foundation 2021).

The Pandemic, Lockdown, Mental Health and Associated Behavioural Problems

As well as its impact upon the mental health of mass publics around the world, the pandemic was also associated with behaviour changes that, in some instances, could be psychologically or physical harmful especially if they persisted over time. Pre-pandemic research had often shown already that these behavioural issues were closely linked to the status of a person's general mental health. As this book has shown, during the novel coronavirus (SARS-CoV-2) pandemic covering the 2020–2021 period, there was evidence of a number of adverse behavioural effects. These were often underpinned by deteriorating psychological health as manifest in reportedly greater than usual stress, anxiety and depression levels in populations. These effects triggered wider concern about contingent behaviour changes such as social isolation and challenges to close interpersonal relationships, deteriorations in intra-family relationships and increased incidences of domestic abuse, greater prevalence of self-harming, increased consumption of alcohol and increased propensity to engage with online gambling.

Evidence has been reviewed about each of these adverse side-effects of the pandemic and more especially of governments' implementation of highly restrictive interventions to slow infection transmission rates. Much of the relevant research, however, was published on the back of quick-turnaround studies aimed at providing timely data to guide policy in a crisis setting. This meant that the evidence produced by this research was based on the measurement of short-term effects of the pandemic and pandemic-related behavioural restrictions. Going forward, it is important to assess whether they might be long-term side-effects of the pandemic crisis that persist long after the pandemic has been deemed to be over. In this chapter, a search has been undertaken to find longitudinal studies – albeit still relatively short-term ones – that might provide indications about what to expect.

Longitudinal data from British participants that examined the mental health effects of the pandemic and the knock-on effects of psychological distress, anxiety and depression on specific behaviour patterns indicated health behaviour could suffer as well as mental state (Villadsen et al., 2021). In particular, among some people, the quality of diet declined, alcohol consumption increased and sleep was disturbed. The effects on sleep were strongest, while effects on alcohol consumption were statistically weak even though significant. Changes in these behaviours were already known to be linked to mental health state before the pandemic, but grew worse during the first national lockdown from March to June 2020. Further soundings, in late summer, when many lockdown restrictions had been lifted, showed that behavioural problems had returned mostly to pre-pandemic levels, the one exception being sleep disturbances. This research confirmed that mental health is important to health behaviour and that both suffered during the pandemic. With many behavioural problems, however, there were also signs that they will improve over time if severe behaviour restrictions imposed by governments during national crises do not persist for too long.

Plotting the Psychological Problems of the Future and Their Solutions

In order to understand longer-term behavioural trends and, within the context of the COVID-19 pandemic, the post-pandemic challenges that lie ahead, data collected longitudinally can be most helpful. Longitudinal studies entail repeated data collection exercises with the same sample of people over time. These exercises might involve asking the participants to complete questionnaires about their beliefs, attitudes, experiences, behaviour and physical or mental well-being at different times. They make take the form of repeat interviews with participants from which these kinds of data can be obtained. They might also entail repeated observations of their behaviour made independent of any direct research-participant interaction. Sometimes, a combination of these methods might be used. The key feature is that specific participants are uniquely identified at each stage of the research. This means that as well as examining data conducted at each collection point, the researchers can also join together data collected at different time points to monitor and measure any changes in participants' behaviours, worldviews and personal status.

Longitudinal data can help to develop trends defined by the directions in which the psychological state of individuals have changed over time and therefore might continue to change in the future. One such study focused on people's psychological health is the COVID-19 Psychological Well-being Study (Armour et al., 2021). This survey was designed to study the impacts of COVID-19 in people across the United Kingdom. Although its sample was not nationally representative, its construction was guided in terms of its demographic and social profiles by adult population profiles derived from the United Kingdom Census. Once recruited, the cohort of participants engaged in data collection exercises every week or month. The aim was to produce a database yielding guidance to future clinical assessment procedures as the country lifted itself out of its pandemic restrictions and its population sought to return their lives as near to pre-pandemic normal as possible.

During the pandemic evidence emerged from multiple sources that the public's psychological health had been adversely impacted by the wide array of restrictions on their everyday behaviours (Zaninotto et al., 2022). These restrictions persisted in many communities with little or no let-up for well over a year. In some settings, there was temporary respite as some restrictions were lifted when COVID-19 cases fell away only to be re-introduced when new waves of rising infection levels occurred. It was anticipated by this project's researchers that anxiety and depression would become more pervasive. Some people would, of course, be more seriously affected than others by these symptoms. There would be already vulnerable individuals for whom the stresses of lockdown were intolerable. Even formerly healthy people might be expected to exhibit a dip in their psychological well-being when their jobs or studies were placed under threat, when they were starved of access to their usual social support networks, and when most forms of entertainment, leisure and distraction were closed off. Deterioration of the psychological state of many people could become so acute that they would be unable to return to "normal" even if they wanted to.

There should be no surprises here. Valuable insights about their psychological impacts on whole populations had been gleaned from research into earlier pandemics. Just within the 21st century (that is the previous 20 years leading up to the COVID-19 outbreak), other diseases which included SARS which was first seen in China in 2003, MERS (Middle East Respiratory Syndrome) which initially broke out in Saudi Arabia in 2012, and H1N1 (Swine) flu which was first noticed in Mexico in April 2009 all triggered local steps designed to control its spread.

In all these cases, psychological distress was especially likely to be reported by front-line healthcare workers, those who had been placed in quarantine and survivors of these diseases and their families (Maunder, 2004; Tsang et al., 2004; Wu et al., 2005; Gardner & Moallef, 2015; Brooks et al., 2020). In respect of COVID-19, early findings recorded similar significant psychological impacts in members of the general population (Qiu et al., 2020; Wang et al., 2020). These impacts most usually took the form of increased levels of anxiety and depression.

The Psychological Wellbeing Study also collected data from its participants about their compliance with their government's behavioural advice and restrictions and their concerns about some of the restrictive measures that had been imposed. This questioning also took account of public confidence in the government and in the efficacy of the interventions being made to control the spread of COVID-19.

This book has not examined compliance. This is the focus of a sister volume (*Psychology of Behaviour Restrictions and Public Compliance in the Pandemic: Lessons from COVID-19*). Nonetheless, the interventions and compliance with them are relevant here because they could also trigger collateral damage. The placement of severe restrictions on what people could do as well as on why they could or could not do certain things created a general psychological climate among communities that could contribute to a general deterioration in a population's psychological health. The worry of becoming infected, anxiety about losing one's job, denial of physical access to family members even if they were very sick and the sheer boredom of having little to do because so much of society was closed down represented a suite of stressors that all came together as a "perfect storm" of behavioural restrictions. The psychological integrity of many individuals was put under great strain. This, in turn, could trigger frustration that undermined social relationships with those with whom people found themselves incarcerated for far greater periods than would normally be the case. On occasions, this frustration could result in behaviourally unhealthy or even destructive responses (Blakey & Abramowitz, 2017; Asmundson & Taylor, 2020; Jungman & Witthoft, 2020).

Another longitudinal study was launched as soon as the first United Kingdom lockdown was implemented. The COVID-19 and Mental Health was run by the COVID-19 Psychological Research Consortium of researchers from the University of Sheffield, Ulster University, University College London, Royal Holloway and Birkbeck College and Maynooth University. An initial sample of 2000 people aged 18+ were recruited within 52 days of the first case of COVID-19 being identified in the United Kingdom during the week beginning 23rd March which was also the date when the British Prime Minister Boris Johnson asked people to stay home except for essential purposes. The Consortium released baseline results in March 2020 (COVID-19 Psychological Research Consortium (C19PRC), 2020).

At this time, initial findings showed fairly to very extensive knowledge of the most common symptoms of COVID-19. Virtually everybody (92–93%) recognised coughing, difficulty breathing and fever as major tell-tale symptoms. The clear majority of respondents noted tiredness (69%) and muscle aches and pains (65% and a sore throat (58% as other common symptoms.

In terms of transmission, the highest risk behaviours were: people coughing and sneezing (94%), people touching each other (89%) and touching surfaces (89%) and breathing the air in confined spaces (72%). Infection risk could be reduced by washing your hands regularly and thoroughly (90%) and by maintaining a distance of one metre between yourself and other people (76%). Many respondents said they were covering their nose when coughing or sneezing (91%) and many were washing their hands (78%) and surfaces at home (82%). During this early stage in the pandemic, however, only a few (17%) said they wore face masks. It is perhaps worth noting that initial guidance offered by the government in March 2020 focused mostly on hand and surface hygiene and greater consciousness about face touching rather than face covering. On a scale of 0–100 there was an average risk score of 48 of getting COVID in the next three months or even in the next month. There was an average score of 44 for getting infected by it in the next six months.

One of the early behavioural reactions observed just before and just after implementation of the first pandemic lockdown in the United Kingdom was panic buying of specified commodities where it was believed that supply chains would cease operating. The initial soundings taken by this survey provided only modest evidence of excess purchasing although a few had said they had bought more dried foods (31%) tinned food (30%), toilet rolls (29%) and hand sanitiser (28%). Further analysis of early buying behaviour in the United Kingdom alongside a comparison sample from the Republic of Ireland found that around three-quarters of the people questioned admitted to over-purchase of a range of commodities. This behaviour was most likely to occur, however, among better off households with dependent children, where householders were also generally more anxious and more paranoid (Bentall et al., 2020).

Being quarantined is an unpleasant experience. It can, for some people, trigger severe psychological reactions including anxiety, stress and depression. These effects can set in amongst the most vulnerable individuals within weeks of lockdown-style interventions. One study from India showed significant increases in depression prevalence (from 23–38%), anxiety prevalence (18–27%) and stress prevalence (9–12%) between weeks two and three of lockdown. These rates were considerably higher than pre-pandemic levels (Pandey et al., 2020). As further evidence indicated, increased stress and anxiety caused by COVID-19 and the interventions implemented to slow its spread caused some already vulnerable individuals and households to experience other behavioural changes including increased domestic violence, alcohol consumption and other risky behaviour such as gambling. Such evidence showed that such vulnerable groups need special attention during a health crisis on this scale.

There was evidence of deterioration in mental health and well-being among British people during March, April and May 2020 followed by some improvement from July 2020 and stabilisation of these problems during August and September 2020. The proportion of adults that reported clinically significant levels of psychological distress increased from 21% in 2019 to 30% by April 2020, a few weeks into the first national lockdown. By September, however, this figure declined to pre-pandemic levels (21%) (Daly & Robinson, 2021). Other research reported similar figures for early onset anxiety and depression during the pandemic (Shevlin et al., 2020).

Further British research also reported increases in the prevalence of anxiety, depression, stress and other associated symptoms such as loneliness and disturbed sleep with subsequent recovery on some though not all symptoms (Fancourt et al., 2021; Zaninotto et al., 2022). Fluctuations in public risk perceptions and fears about COVID-19 tended to coincide with periods of national lockdown. When restrictions were tightened, the public became more concerned. When they were relaxed, so too did people's anxieties about the virus. Further research will be needed going forward to establish which collateral effects were immediate responses to the pandemic and which were more persistent while also identifying population sub-groups that displayed the greatest susceptibility to the manifold cognitive, emotional and behavioural side-effects identified in this book.

References

Armour, C., McGlinchey, E., Butter, S. McAloney-Kocaman, & McPherson, K. E. (2021). The COVID-19 psychological wellbeing study: Understanding the longitudinal psychosocial impact of the COVID-19 pandemic in the UK; a methodological overview paper. *Journal of Psychopathology and Behaviour Assessment*, 43: 174–190. https://doi.org/10.1007/s10862-020-09841-4

Asmundson, G. J., & Taylor, S. (2020). Coronaphobia: Fear and the 2019-nCoV outbreak. *Journal of Anxiety Disorders*, 70: 102196. 10.1016/j.janxdis.2020. 102196

Bahn, G. H. (2020). Coronavirus disease 2019, school closures and children's mental health. *Journal of the Korean Academic and Child and Adolescent Psychiatry*, 31(2): 74–79.

Bentall, R. P., Lloyd, A., Bennett, K., McKay, R., Mason, L., Murphy, J., McBride, O., Hartman, T. K., Gibson-Miller, J., Levita, L., Martinez, A. P., Stocks, T. V. A., Butter, S., Vallières, F., Hyland, P., Karatzias, T., & Shevlin, M. (2020). Pandemic buying: Testing a psychological model of over-purchasing and panic buying using data from the United Kingdom and the Republic of Ireland during the early phase of the COVID-19 pandemic. *PLOS ONE, 16*(1): e0246339. doi:10.1371/journal. pone.0246339

Blakey, S. M. & Abramowitz, J. S. (2017). Psychological predictors of health anxiety in response to the Zika virus. *Journal of Clinical Psychology in Medical Settings*, 24(3–4): 270–278. 10.1007/s10880-017-9514-y

Brooks, S. K., Webster, R. K., Smith, L. E., Woodland, L., Wessely, S., Greenberg, N., & Rubin, G. J. (2020). The psychological impact of quarantine and how to reduce it: Rapid review of the evidence. *The Lancet*, 395(10227): 912–920. 10. 1016/S0140-6736(20)30460-8

Brunier, A., & Drysdale, C. (2022, 2nd March). COVID-19 pandemic triggers 25% increase in prevalence of anxiety and depression worldwide. Geneva, Switzerland: World Health Organization. Retrieved from: https://www.who.int/news/item/02-03-2022-covid-19-pandemic-triggers-25-increase-in-prevalence-of-anxiety-and-depression-worldwide

Carers Trust (2020, July). *My Future, My Feelings, My Family*. Retrieved from: https://carers.org/downloads/what-we-do-section/my-future-my-feelings-my-family.pdf

Conroy, D. & Nicholls, E. (2020, 11th May). All in this together. The Psychologist. Retrieved from: https://thepsychologist.bps.org.uk/all-together

COVID-19 Psychological Research Consortium (C19PRC). (2020). *Initial Research Findings on the COVID-19 and Mental Health in the UK*. Retrieved from https://www.newswise.com/pdf_docs/158566202555665_C19PRC%20wave %201%20initial%20report.pdf

Daly, M. & Robinson, E. (2021, January 14). Longitudinal changes in psychological distress in the UK from 2019 to September 2020 during the COVID-19 pandemic: Evidence from a large nationally representative study. 10.31234/osf.io/mjg72

Fancourt, D., Bu, F., Mak, H. W., & Steptoe, A. (2020). *UK COVID-19 Social Study. Results Release 3*. Retrieved from: https://b6bdcb03–332c-4ff9-8b9d-28f9c957493a.filesusr.com/ugd/3d9db5_13e8d6ef4dd34caf94a7a7b9ae359c95.pdf

Fancourt, D., Steptoe, A., & Bu, F. (2020). Trajectories of depression and anxiety during enforced isolation due to COVID-19: Longitudinal analyses of 59,318 adults in the UK with and without diagnosed mental illness. *medRxiv*. Retrieved from: https://www.medrxiv.org/content/10.1101/2020.06.03.20120923v1

Fancourt, D., Bu, F., Mak, H. W., Paul, E., & Steptoe, A. (2021, 25th March). Covid-19 Social Study: Results Release 32. Department of Behaviour Science and Health, University College London. Retrieved from: https://b6bdcb03–332c-4ff9-8b9d-28f9c957493a.filesusr.com/ugd/3d9db5_c559cf48943940b196853ce33da1e8b2.pdf

Fancourt, D., Steptoe, A., & Bu, F. (2021). Trajectories of anxiety and depressive symptoms during enforced isolation due to COVID-19 in England: A longitudinal observational study. *Lancet Psychiatry*, 8(2): 141–149.

Fegert, J. M., Vitiello, B., Plener, P. L., & Clemens, V. (2020). Challenges and burden of the Coronavirus 2019 (COVID-19) pandemic for child and adolescent mental health: A narrative review to highlight clinical and research needs in the acute phase and the long return to normality. *Child and Adolescent Psychiatry and Mental Health*, 14: 20. 10.1186/s13034-020-00329-3

Gardner, P. J. & Moallef, P. (2015). Psychological impact on SARS survivors: Critical review of the English language literature. *Canadian Psychology*, 56(1): 123–135. 10.1037/a0037973

Holmes, E. A., O'Connor, R. C., Perry, V. H., Tracey, I., Wessely, S., Arseneault, L., Ballard, C., Christensen, H., Cohen Silver, R., Everall, I., Ford, T., John, A., Kabir, T., King, K., Madan, I., Michie, S., Przybylski, A. K., Shafran, R., Sweeney, A., Worthman, C. M., Yardley, L., Cowan, K., Cope, C., Hotopf, M., & Bullmore, E. (2020). Multidisciplinary research priorities for the COVID-19 pandemic: a call for action for mental health science. *Lancet Psychiatry*, 7(6): 547–560. doi: 10.1016/S2215-0366(20)30168-1

Jungmann, S. M. & Witthöft, M. (2020). Health anxiety, cyberchondria, and coping in the current COVID-19 pandemic: Which factors are related to coronavirus anxiety? *Journal of Anxiety Disorders*, 102239. 10.1016/j.janxdis.2020.102239

Kim, A. (2020, 26th November). Young people's anxiety levels neatly doubled during first Covid-19 lockdown, study says. CNN. Retrieved from: https://edition.cnn.com/2020/11/25/health/covid-mental-health-wellness-trnd/index.html

Leigh-Hunt, N., Bagguley, D., Bash, K., Turner, V., Turnbull, S., Valtorta, N., & Caan, W. (2017). An overview of systematic reviews on the public health consequences of social isolation and loneliness. *Public Health*, 152: 157–171. doi: 10.1016/j.puhe.2017.07.035

Liang, L., Ren, H., Cao, R., Hu, Y., Qin, Z., Li, C., & Mei, S. (2020). The effect of COVID-19 on youth mental health. *Psychiatry Quarterly*, 91(3): 841–852. doi: 10.1007/s11126-020-09744-3

Liu, J. J., Bao, Y., Huang, X., Shi, J., & Lu, L. (2020). Mental health considerations for children quarantined because of COVID-19. *Lancet Child and Adolescent Health*, 4(5): 347–349. doi: 10.1016/S2352-4642(20)30096-1

Lucas, M., Nelson, J., & Sims, D. (2020). *Schools' responses to COVID-19: Pupil engagement in remote learning*. Slough, UK: National Foundation for Educational Research. Retrieved from: https://www.nfer.ac.uk/schools-responses-to-covid-19-pupil-engagement-in-remote-learning/

Maunder, R. (2004). The experience of the 2003 SARS outbreak as a traumatic stress among frontline healthcare workers in Toronto: Lessons learned. *Philosophical Transactions of the Royal Society of London Series B: Biological Sciences*, 359(1447): 1117–1125. 10.1098/rstb.2004.1483

Mental Health Foundation (2020). Coronavirus: Mental Health in the Pandemic. Retrieved from https://www.mentalhealth.org/our-work/resarch/coronavirus-mental-health

Mental Health Foundation (2021). Impacts of lockdown on the mental health of children and young people. Retrieved from: https://www.mentalhealth.org.uk/publications/impacts-lockdown-mental-health-children-and-young-people

Pandey, D., Bansal, S., Goyal, S., Garg, A., Sethi, N., Pothiyill, D. I., et al. (2020). Psychological impact of mass quarantine on population during pandemics—The COVID-19 Lock-Down (COLD) study. *PLoS ONE*, 15(10): e0240501. 10.1371/journal.pone.0240501

Pierce, M., McManus, S., Hope, H., Hotopf, M., Ford, T., Hatch, S., John, A., Kontopantelis, E., Webb, R. T., Wessley, S., & Abel, K. (2021). Mental health responses to the COVID-19 pandemic: a latent class trajectory analysis using longitudinal UK data. *Lancet Psychiatry*, 8(7): 610–619. doi: 10.1016/S2215-0366(21)00151-6 Retrieved from: https://papers.ssrn.com/sol3/papers.cfm?abstract_id=3784647

Qiu, J., Shen, B., Zhao, M., Wang, Z., Xie, B., & Xu, Y. (2020). A nationwide survey of psychological distress among Chinese people in the COVID-19 epidemic: implications and policy recommendations. *General Psychiatry*, 33(2): e100213. doi: 10.1136/gpsych-2020-100213. Erratum in: Gen Psychiatr. 2020 Apr 27;33(2):e100213corr1

Saurabk, K. & Ranjan, S. (2020). Compliance and psychological impact of quarantine in children and adolescents due to Covid-19 Pandemic. *Indian Journal of Pediatrics*, 87: 532–536.

Shanks, G. D. & Brundage, J. F. (2012). Pathogenic responses among young adults during the 1918 influenza pandemic. *Emerging infectious diseases*, 18(2): 201–207. 10.3201/eid1802.102042

Shevlin, M., McBride, O., Murphy, J., Gibson-Miller, J., Hartman, T. K., Levita, L., Mason, L., Martinez, A. P., McKay, R., Stocks, T. V. A., Bennett, K. M., Hyland, P., Karatzias, T., & Bentall., R. P. (2020). Anxiety, depression, traumatic stress and COVID-19 related anxiety in the UK general population during the COVID-19 pandemic. *British Journal of Psychology Open*, 6(6): e125. doi:10.1192/bjo.2020.109

Sprang, G. & Silman, M. (2013). Posttraumatic stress disorder in parents and youth after health-related disasters. *Disaster Medicine and Public Health Preparedness*, 7(1): 105–110.

Stevenson, B. L., Dvorak, R. D., Kramer, M. P., Peterson, R. S., Dunn, M. E., Leary, A. V., & Pinto, D. (2019). Within- and between-person associations from mood to alcohol consequences: The mediating role of enhancement and coping drinking motives. *Journal of Abnormal Psychology*, 128980: 813.

Symonds, J. E. (2020, 16th April). Positive pandemic? *The Psychologist*. Retrieved from: https://thepsychologist.bps.org.uk/positive-pandemic

Tsang, H. W., Scudds, R. J., & Chan, E. Y. (2004). Psychosocial impact of SARS. *Emerging Infectious Diseases*, 10(7): 1326–1327. 10.3201/eid1007.040090

Villadsen, A., Patalay, P., & Bann, D. (2021). Mental health in relation to changes in sleep, exercise, alcohol and diet during the COVID-19 pandemic: examination of four UK cohort studies. *Psychological Medicine*, 1–10. doi: 10.1017/S0033291721004657 Epub ahead of print. Retrieved from: https://www.medrxiv.org/content/10.1101/2021.03.26.21254424v2

Vindegaard, N. & Benros, M. E. (2020). COVID-19 pandemic and mental health consequences: Systematic review of the current evidence. *Brain, Behaviour and Immunity*, 89: 531–542. doi: 10.1016/j.bbi.2020.05.048

Waite, P., Moltrecht, B., McElroy, E., & Cresseell, C. (2020). *Covid-19 Worries, Parent/carer Stress and Support Needs, by Child Special Education Needs and Parent-status*

Status. Oxford, UK: The Co-Space Study. Retrieved from: https://emergingminds.org.uk/wp-content/uploads/2020/05/Co-SPACE-report-02_03-05-20.pdf

Wang, G., Zhang, Y., Zhao, J., Zhang, J., & Jiang, F. (2020). Mitigate the effects of home confinement on children during the COVID-19 outbreak. *Lancet*, 395 (10228): 945–947.

Wang, Y., Xu, B., Zhao, G., Cao, R., He, X., & Fu, S. (2011). Is quarantine related to immediate negative psychological consequences during the 2009 H1N1 epidemic? *General Hospital* Psychiatry, 33(1): 75–77.

Wu, K. K., Chan, S. K., & Ma, T. M. (2005). Posttraumatic stress, anxiety, and depression in survivors of severe acute respiratory syndrome (SARS). *Journal of Traumatic Stress*, 18(1): 39–42. 10.1002/jts.20004

Xie, X., Xue, Q., Zhou, Y., Zhu, K., Liu, Q., Zhang, J., & Song, R. (2020). Mental health status among children in home confinement during the coronavirus disease 2019 outbreak in Hubei Province, China. *JAMA Pediatrics*, 174(9): 898–900. doi: 10.1001/jamapediatrics.2020.1619

Youth Link Scotland (2020). *Lockdown Lowdown: What Young People in Scotland are Thinking about COVID-19*. The Scottish Youth Parliament, Youth Link Scotland and Young Scot. Retrieved from: https://www.youthlinkscotland.org/media/4486/lockdown-lowdown-final-report.pdf

Zaninotto, P., Iob, E., Demakakos, P., & Steptoe, A. (2022). Immediate and Longer-Term Changes in the Mental Health and Well-being of Older Adults in England During the COVID-19 Pandemic. *JAMA psychiatry*, 79(2), 151–159. *JAMA psychiatry*, 79(2): 151–159. https://doi.org/10.1001/jamapsychiatry.2021.3749

Index

Page numbers followed by t indicate tables

Printed in the United States
by Baker & Taylor Publisher Services